Smooth Muscle Cells in Atherosclerosis

Monographs on Atherosclerosis

Vol. 2

Editors:
Otakar J. Pollak, Dover, Delaware, USA
Henry S. Simms, Rockleigh, New Jersey, USA
John Esben Kirk, St. Louis, Missouri, USA

S. Karger · Basel · München · Paris · London · New York · Sydney

Smooth Muscle Cells in Atherosclerosis

J. C. GEER and M. DARIA HAUST
Department of Pathology, The Ohio State University, Columbus, Ohio,
and The University of Western Ontario, London, Ontario

With 27 figures

19 72

S. Karger · Basel · München · Paris · London · New York · Sydney

Supported by Grants HE-02549 and 11896 from The National Heart Institute, US Public Health Service, The Harker Fund, and Grants-in-Aid of Research MT-1037 from The Medical Research Council of Canada and T-11 from The Ontario Heart Foundation, Toronto, Ontario, Canada.

Monographs on Atherosclerosis

Vol. 1

O. J. POLLAK (Dover, Delaware): Tissue Cultures.
XII + 143 p., 28 fig. comprising 49 black and white and 32 color illustrations, 9 tab., 1969

S. Karger · Basel · München · Paris · London · New York · Sydney
Arnold-Böcklin-Strasse 25, CH-4011 Basel (Switzerland)

Printed in Switzerland by Buchdruckerei Effingerhof AG, Brugg
Blocks: Steiner & Co., Basel

Dedicated to our respective families

Contents

Acknowledgements

The authors wish to thank Mrs. Lee Bangs and Mrs. Mary-Lou Duffy for competent typing of the manuscript in its various stages; and Mrs. Maria Oteruelo, Mrs. Joanna Egli and Mrs. Margaret Davis for assistance in assembling the references.

Illustrations

The authors have not attempted to illustrate all the morphological features of normal and abnormal arteries for obvious reasons. We have attempted to select a series of micrographs that illustrate the more important points and have arranged these in the order of an atlas. The order in which these illustrations are arranged is normal, diffuse, intimal thickening, mural thrombosis, fatty streak, and fibrous plaque. The legends to the illustrations of course represent the opinion of the authors and others may choose to interpret these differently. Regardless of differences in opinion for interpretation we have tried to depict representative cells of the types that are found in human arteries.

Preface

Following the presentation concerning the role of smooth muscle cells in atherosclerosis at a recent Gordon Conference (Providence Heights, Washington, June 1969), one of the participants watching the 'fiery' reactions and arguments of the discussants, remarked publicly: 'I don't understand all this commotion and heated discussion on the subject of smooth muscle cells, as if they were discovered only recently. These cells have been with us for a long time and were often referred to by many "old" German histologists and pathologists.' In general, this statement is applicable to innumerable so-called recent 'discoveries', and if one checks the older literature, including the German and French writings, one finds that most of the 'new' observations were thoroughly investigated, even though with much simpler tools than those in use today, and reported in detail many decades or even a century ago.

Nevertheless, the statement quoted above is correct only out of context, and it is doubtful that when made it was realized that the subject was atherosclerosis. For, as far as the role of the smooth muscle cells in atherosclerosis is concerned, our knowledge is very new indeed, as it evolved, at first slowly, over the past fifteen years only. In the last five years we have witnessed an enormous burst of activities with respect to smooth muscle cells, both in the investigation of human and experimental atherosclerosis. Attesting to the recent surge of activities in this field is the fact that the present authors abandoned the idea of writing this monograph in 1963 (following the International Symposium on the Evolution of the Atherosclerotic Plaque held in Chicago, March 28–29, 1963) [137] because there would not have been but at the most a handful of centers where work on the role of smooth muscle cells in atherosclerosis was going on – quite a meager substrate for a monograph. When approached regarding the writing of this monograph, the authors decided that perhaps this is the last opportunity to put together meaningful information on the subject, as the field had mushroomed to such an extent that the task of reviewing this field soon will become impossible.

A refreshing aspect with a human touch of the development in the field under consideration is the fact that studies of smooth muscle cells (in atherosclerosis) stretched from the South to the North across the North American continent to embrace two centers of independent thought, and effected lasting friendships between the investigators involved. It is, therefore, quite appropriate that the representatives from each center (originally New Orleans, Louisiana, and Kingston, Ontario) collaborated in the present endeavor. Were it not for the fact that the five people originally involved reside at present at five different locations, this 'opus' would have been the outcome of writing of five people. For reasons of expediency, there are only two writers involved. Nevertheless, the authors consider that this monograph represents the outcome of inspiration and work also of the three other investigators and friends, Dr. Robert H. More, McGill University, Montreal, Canada, Dr. Henry C. McGill, jr., The University of Texas Medical School, San Antonio, Texas, and Dr. Jack P. Strong, Louisiana State University Medical Center, New Orleans, Louisiana.

I. Introductory Remarks and Terminology

This short monograph has two aims: (a) to collect, collate and integrate data on the subject of smooth muscle cells in atherosclerosis that have emerged in contemporary times; and (b) to review the 'old' literature on some aspects of the same subject in detail in order to correct the misquotations, confusions and at times a downright dilettante perpetuation of wrong information.

In selecting the mode of approach as well as the content for the present monograph, the authors made the following arbitrary decisions in order that attention be focused on the subject matter as sharply as possible:

1. Since atherosclerosis affects large elastic and medium-size muscular arteries, the review and data presentation is limited to these two types of arteries only. Occasionally, when certain information considered to be of importance pertains to other vessels (small arteries, veins), it is quoted – assuming that it may have some bearing also upon the problem discussed. Moreover, in view of the desire to concentrate largely on human atherosclerosis, data are being presented in detail whenever available in man; work on normal arterial structure and experimental atherosclerosis in animals is included in the main either because no data are (or can be!) available in man, or when they are at variance with those in man.

2. The role of smooth muscle cells in atherosclerosis can be viewed only in the context of the organ affected and the disease process itself. This necessitates a relatively detailed discussion on the subject of normal structure and some functional aspects of arteries (as delineated under paragraph 1 above) as a basis for the understanding of the pathological process in which the major cellular element of the entire arterial wall, i.e., the smooth muscle cell, plays an important role. Thus, a short chapter on the structure of normal arterial wall precedes the deliberations on the role of smooth muscle cells in atherosclerosis, as does also a chapter on diffuse intimal thickening. The latter is set separately to emphasize that this diffuse intimal change is *not* a part of atherosclerotic process, even if it may have some bearing upon the latter. Finally, an abbreviated morphological account on all forms of athero-

sclerotic lesions was included for the same (above) reasons, even if at present the role of smooth muscle cells in some of these has not been delineated or even established.

3. The chapter entitled, 'Identification of Cells in Atherosclerotic Lesions – A Historical Review', is by design devoted to a narrow segment as specified in the opening remarks of that section, and the reviewing is carried only until the time when facts (as accepted today) were established. Beyond this period and the narrow topic selected, pertinent data are reviewed in the other individual sections.

4. Not all or even most publications entirely or partially devoted to the field under consideration are quoted in this monograph. Care was taken with respect to only two extremes, i.e., to insure on one hand that the work of 'pioneers' and key additions to it be quoted, and on the other that publications based on data that do not appear sound, be omitted. Beyond that no firm rule could be exercised. When a given publication affirmed only the observations already made, it was usually not included, unless it strengthened the original position that was regarded by others as contentious. Similarly, the quotation of work on various species is not complete; it was included where differences between species should be stressed. And finally, some work is not quoted because the publications on the subject had mushroomed to such an extent that the authors simply may not be aware of all the work published.

5. No attempt is made to arbitrate the discrepancies of data pertaining to the measurement of structures studied by electron microscopy, since it is well known that artifacts affecting the size of these are introduced by tissue processing and the latter varies from one method to another, or even with the same method in different hands. In some instances, measurements are omitted by design, because very small or very large dimensions are particularly subject to errors; in other instances, a range of, rather than precisely defined measurements are quoted.

This monograph concerns itself clearly with the smooth muscle cells in atherosclerotic lesions and is entitled accordingly. It may thus appear superfluous to devote, no matter how small, a section to definitions and terminology, other than perhaps to additional areas of the monograph that may require specifications. The latter is, however, not necessary, and the substance of this section relates solely to the smooth muscle cells, because the authors consider it rather important to voice their opinion against 'splitting' and the use of jargon that has crept into the scientific language. The objection is being voiced not only for 'purity' or academic reason; as will be argued, the flourishing terminology is not only unnecessary but, more importantly, partly incorrect and quite vague.

It will be documented in this monograph that the cells of atherosclerotic lesions are defined in morphological and functional terms as smooth muscle cells: the shapes of the nucleus and the cell itself conform in broad terms to those of other smooth muscle cells; the cells contain fibrils whose special staining reactions and electron microscopic appearance are identical to those of other myofilaments; the cells are wrapped by a PAS-positive basement membrane, possess a variable number of pinocytotic vesicles, and contain contractile proteins that by immunological methods are similar, if not identical, to those of smooth muscle cells in other organs (i.e., uterus). Thus, it should matter little that there may be other features distinguishing these cells from their 'sisters' elsewhere. After all, the cells that populate the gastrointestinal tract are morphologically different, e.g., than those of the arterial media, ureteral wall, or the uterus. If we were thus to refer to the cells in atherosclerotic lesions as to myointimal cells, as some would have us do, for the sake of consistency we would have to speak of myo-medial, myo-uterine, myo-intestinal, myo-vesicular, myo-ureteral and so on, cells!

Others would have us refer to these cells as myo-endothelial cells in considering the purportedly single origin of these cells from the endothelium – the latter is still an extremely controversial matter. But even if it were generally accepted that the endothelium were the sole source of origin, why not – in the same vein – indicate by an appropriate name the origin of other smooth muscle cells?

The strongest objection to the usage of the above terminology (myo-intimal or myo-endothelial) is made on the basis that both are somewhat incorrect, as the prefixed 'myo-' implies only 'muscular in nature' without specification whether smooth or striated muscle is meant. Thus, purportedly attempting to pinpoint these cells, an error is being committed to refer to them in even more vague, unspecified and almost incorrect terms.

On the other hand, the term 'modified smooth muscle cells', as it applies to cells in certain forms or stages of atherosclerotic lesions (and under many experimental conditions), is quite acceptable. These cells are recognizable as smooth muscle cells, but lack one or several of their characteristic features and thus some criteria for identification.

To those who consider all forms of these cells in the context of dynamics (whether this be in normal or atherosclerotic intima), *as most pathologists do,* they represent smooth muscle cells that adapted themselves structurally as well as functionally to the environment they were designated to live in.

II. Identification of Cells in Atherosclerotic Lesions – A Historical Review

Inherent in any attempt at reviewing the 'old' literature is a twofold danger; the review may be carried out for the sake of 'reviewing' and traditional completeness, and consists of endless enumeration of statements made by our forefathers in science – without direction to, or 'backbone' of this amassed information, and in the end nobody knows what is being reviewed. Alternatively, some reviews of 'old' literature have the air of a smug presumption purporting to document how little was known before the modern (and often one's own) enlightment in science!

Nevertheless, historical reviews are often not only desirable but necessary in rectifying wrong assumptions thus establishing facts, and when approached critically and in a 'directional' fashion may be helpful in focusing upon problems to be solved and a path that future research should pursue. With the above in mind we have chosen to concentrate our attention upon reviewing the following:

Documentation of the initial work and establishing the fact that smooth muscle cells are *the* cellular elements involved in the inception and progression of atherosclerotic lesions in man and experimental animals by undergoing degenerative or proliferative changes; thus, they are an important factor in both the fatty dots and streaks and in fibrous plaques.

However, even the above intention to limit and define the area of review carries with it an inherent difficulty which pertains to the review of work before 1960 and particularly that reported until the mid-thirties, as it is seldom possible to assess at what 'developmental' level the described lesions were. Most investigators refer to 'early changes', and 'later these lesions show', often without specifying the gross appearance of these lesions, or whether 'later' was regarded as the endpoint, or an assumed next step in the development. It is therefore extremely difficult to compare the findings of one investigator with those of others. Moreover, the experimental methods and species used vary so widely that one wonders whether comparisons under those diverse circumstances with respect to a specific component, i.e., the cell, may be meaningful at all. How can one compare lesions produced even by the same compound, but by various doses or administered at different time intervals or over a different period with each other? One should review *these differences* rather than similarities more carefully than anyone attempted to date, if interpretation of histogenesis of lesions is to throw some light on the pathogenesis of the disease. For example, BAILEY [14, pp. 76–77] reported on the results of feeding rabbits with egg yolk: 'In rabbits 12 and 16 which were fed longer than any of the other rabbits but with smaller doses, the aortic lesions differed somewhat from those in the other rabbits. While the intimal lesions were of the same character (as those found in animals fed larger doses) with many large fat-filled cells, the intimal thickening was not nearly as pronounced, fibrosis was slight, and areas of degeneration with the deposit of cholesterol were not found. The media, however, was more markedly affected than in the rabbits receiving larger doses for a shorter period.' When one takes the trouble to check the doses of rabbits 12 and 16, one finds that one received twice as much as the other in an approximately the same length of time (68 egg yolks in 138 days versus 32½ egg yolks in 134 days). This example from BAILEY's work was chosen because it poses at once at least three vital questions: Within what limits (of doses administered) is an investigator justified to 'pool' his observations; should the pooling be done on the basis of the similarity of the lesions produced rather than doses administered; and finally, how should these observations be interpreted? In other words, in the final analysis there is very little value in any reviewing unless there is a component of *evaluation* in this reviewing, e.g., do BAILEY's data regarding the above findings suggest that the intake of 'smaller' (what is the critical point?) doses of egg yolk is not very harmful to the artery because there is no cellular degeneration, no cholesterol (presumably extracellular) deposition and little fibrosis; or, alternatively, is it more harmful because the underlying media was affected more markedly than in the animal series on larger doses? And do these experiments suggest that the intimal cells can 'handle' a certain amount of lipids (derived from the egg yolk), i.e., they accumulate fats, but can metabolize these (what is the critical point?) either continuously or in the intervals when egg yolk was omitted from feeding (both rabbits received yolk daily with the exception of either 'an occasional interval' or 'an occasional interval of a few days')?

Obviously, in view of an enormous body of information that accumulated even in the rather narrow areas selected for reviewing, an attempt at reviewing in terms as exemplified above would be impossible in a monograph of this, rather limited, size. Nevertheless, the above example of 'analyzing when reviewing' was intended to underline the necessity of a component of analysis in each review. The presence of one or another cell in atherosclerotic lesions is interesting, and determining the identity of each necessary for a true scientific endeavor. But for pathologists, it must imply beyond that something more; it must convey a glimpse or a frame of a dynamic process which we hope to understand in order to learn how to prevent it. And thus any reviewing of facts must be accompanied always by a question: 'What does this mean?'

It has been observed by many investigators concerned with the initial analysis of atherosclerotic lesions at the end of the last and in the beginning of this century that basically, there are cells that contain fat and those that are fat-free, the latter being associated with proliferation of connective tissues in fibrous plaques. The nature and derivation of these cells as well as their relation to each other (if at all) had been a matter of controversy until our times, and indeed, their true identity was established unequivocally only in recent years largely with the help of electron microscopy.

The Fat-Containing Cells

These cells had always been recognized as the main feature of the yellow dots and streaks, but were observed in smaller numbers also in older lesions between the dense connective tissue fibers, and in the other, more controversial lesions of atherosclerosis (see chapt. V on early lesions). These cells were variously referred to as foam cells, lipoid cells, xanthoma cells, 'cholinester'-phagocytes, or 'lutein-like' cells. Three different cell types had been implicated in the phenomenon of intracellular lipid accumulation and whereas some investigators insisted on a 'monolithic' approach, others considered that in atherosclerosis more than one cell type may contain lipids. The lipid-containing cells were thought to be either mononuclear phagocytes, endothelial cells, or other local intimal cells (fibroblasts, mesenchymal cells, smooth muscle cells).

Mononuclear Phagocytes (Macrophages)

In 1935, DUFF [55] discussed the three possible sources of the mononuclear phagocytes in the atherosclerotic lesions: (1) The cells could arise from a multiplication of wandering mononuclear phagocytes present in the intima prior to the appearance of lipids (and phagocytize the fat *in situ*), a theory favored by him and many other investigators; (2) the foam cells could have migrated from the media, a view not supported by either him or the observations of others; and (3) the cells may represent macrophages that enter the intima from the lumen. According to ANITSCHKOW [8], small lymphocytic (or lymphoid) cells should be added to the last category since in his experience not only did he observe frequently lymphoid and monocytic cells 'to invade' the aortic wall directly from the lumen, but in addition, he found all conceivable transitional forms between the small lymphocytic and monocytic cells on the one hand, and on the other the large lipid-containing cells. Similar derivation of foam cells in the intima of small arteries of organs exposed to radiation was proposed by SHEEHAN [250].

The matter of the possible derivation of the lipid-containing cells in atherosclerosis from circulating mononuclear cells (phagocytes) became more complex and controversial when LEARY published his work [161], for he believed that the cells invading the intima from the lumen were already fat-containing, specifically cholesterol ester, and that this event actually heralded the inception of an atherosclerotic lesion. According to him, hypercholesterolemia (whether it be experimental or in man) burdens primarily the hepatic cells with accumulation of cholesterol esters above the normal threshold. Subsequently, the esters are removed by Kupffer cells of the liver (and in adrenals by analogous cells). These fat-containing derivatives of the reticuloendothelial system, having entered the blood stream, pass through the lung 'filter' and enter selectively the arterial intima... 'apparently due to a positive chemotaxis which is selective for cholesterol. Stresses favor the localization of the cells' (verbatim quotation) [161, p. 539]. In terms of the definition of a positive chemotaxis, this statement is largely incorrect, and, moreover, inconsistent with LEARY's own insistence that no (extracellular) cholesterol other than 'accidental' is present in the intima prior to the invasion of these cholesterol esters-bearing cells. In support of his interpretation of this pathogenesis of atherosclerotic lesions, he quotes ASCHOFF's [10] statement that '... a certain number of reticuloendothelial cells or blood histiocytes pass the filter of the lungs and the heart and enter the general circulation', as well as the firm conviction expressed by KLOTZ [151] that in early atherosclerotic lesions fat was first intracellular. Neither of the aforementioned statements could be taken, however, to support LEARY's theory that the blood histiocytes enter the intima already in the form of foam cells. LEARY's way of thinking did not gain support, despite the attempts of GORDON [92] to explain the phenomenon of intimal invasion by lipophages by a different property than 'chemotaxis'. He assumed that lipophages being lighter than other blood corpuscles leave the axial stream and enter the peripheral zone of the blood current during diastole; thus, they come to lie close to endothelium enabling the process of emigration. Another modification of LEARY's version was advanced by RANNIE and DUGUID [228] who believed on the basis of their observations in experimental atherosclerosis in rabbits that, indeed, the foam cells were derived from the circulating blood but they did not invade the intima by simply penetrating through the endothelial lining; rather, clumps of these foam cells adhered to the arterial wall and endothelium grew over them, so that they became incorporated into the wall in a fashion similar to thrombus incorporation. POOLE and FLOREY concluded in 1958 that their own work [224] provided evidence in support of the belief and work of others [55, 182] that macrophages undergo mitosis in atherosclerotic lesions and may thus be the source of foam cells, and whereas macrophages may arrive via blood stream, they do not necessarily take up lipoid material until after gaining attachment to the endothelium. However, they questioned whether a reasonable explanation could be provided for the phenomenon that macrophages, but no other cells, adhered to the endothelium in the areas of lesion. They also refute the suggestion of RANNIE and DUGUID [228] that the fat-containing cells are incorporated by endothelial overgrowth, as in their experimental work no morphological changes that usually accompany endothelial proliferation (occurrence of endothelial giant and multinucleated cells, the presence of nuclei of varying size and staining quality) could be observed.

To test the derivation of fat-containing cells in atherosclerotic lesions from reticuloendothelial system at distant, i.e., extra-arterial sites, experiments aiming at labelling the system either prior to, or following experimental hypercholesterolemia in rabbits, were carried out by several groups of investigators. KUNTZ and SULKIN [155] administered either India ink or lithium carmine intravenously to hypercholesterolemic rabbits, and observed pigment granules in visceral phagocytes, but none in the foam cells of the atherosclerotic lesions. Considering that the labelling of reticuloendothelial system prior to the inception of atherosclerotic lesions may be of prime importance in testing the theory, SIMONTON and GOFMAN [258] administered colloidal thorium dioxide to rabbits prior to cholesterol feeding. Thorium-containing phagocytes in the liver and spleen engulfed India ink injected 24 hours before death. The amount of radioactivity in the atherosclerotic lesions was very low, and the investigators concluded that the fat-containing macrophages derived from distant reticuloendothelial sites did not contribute significantly to the foam cells of atherosclerotic lesions in rabbits. Later,

HARRIS [99] induced in rabbits hypercholesterolemia for two weeks prior to injecting India ink at weekly intervals, while the animals continued on cholesterol-rich diet. The reticuloendothelial cells of all rabbits were laden with carbon, whereas pigment-containing phagocytes were not found in atherosclerotic lesions. Nevertheless, these various 'labelling' experiments do not provide proof that foam cells in atherosclerotic lesions are not derived from fat-containing reticuloendothelial cells of distant sites. All that can be stated on the basis of these studies is that labelled pigmented reticuloendothelial cells are not found in the lesions; this may only indicate that either the pigment-laden cells became more sessile and do not migrate with ease, or that even when migrating, they have lost their affinity (as postulated by LEARY) for the arterial intima or ability to penetrate the endothelial lining.

Recently, there was an attempt at revival of the since largely dismissed theory of LEARY, in still another modified form. Stimulated by electron microscopic observations that foam cells penetrated endothelium [264] and that numerous circulating lipophages preceded the development of atherosclerosis in the rat [257, 271], a study was undertaken to compare the ultrastructure of the circulating lipophages and the lipid-containing cells in atherosclerotic lesions of hyperlipemic rats. It was concluded that the foam cells in lesions were derived, indeed, from the circulating lipophages that penetrated the arterial endothelium, but once in the intima, these cells continued to accumulate fat *in situ* [175]. This attempt at compromising the two extreme views, i.e., that the foam cells originating at distant sites (liver, adrenal) enter the intima from the lumen as such on the one hand, and on the other that they result from an *in situ* phagocytosis by macrophages, has not received much support, either.

A general consensus of opinion that some foam cells are derived from mononuclear phagocytes was reached in the years 1960–1962 on the basis of electron microscopic examination of experimental [214] and human [75, 111] atherosclerotic lesions. These mononuclear phagocytes may originate either from the circulating blood or wandering tissue histiocytes, but they phagocytize fat *in situ*, i.e., in the intima; however, this is not the initial step in the evolution of the lesion as it represents a sequence to an earlier change involving the native cells, nor do all foam cells originate from the macrophages (see below). Just what proportion of foam cells is derived from mononuclear phagocytes has not been determined; some believe even now, on the basis of histoenzymatic and histochemical studies, that all foam cells in the lesions are of macrophagic derivation [17].

Endothelial Cells

There had been largely two schools of thought on the subject of endothelial cells as a source of foam cells in atherosclerotic lesions that may be formulated as follows: (1) Lipid accumulates in the endothelial cells and these migrate into the intima, or (2) endothelial cells proliferate and migrate into the intima where they acquire lipid and thereby assume the appearance of foam cells. Furthermore, there is difference of opinion whether in either case lipid is actively phagocytized by the endothelial cells, or whether it accumulates as an expression of degeneration (fatty metamorphosis).

That lipid droplets may accumulate in the endothelial cells in atherosclerosis has been documented by many investigators [4, 6, 15, 75, 101, 131, 212, 214, 224, 246, 281, 286], but the extent to which this may occur had been questioned by some authorities in the field [56]. Those who maintain that the presence of fat in the endothelium represents phagocytosis could be supported by the demonstration of the phagocytic property of the vascular endothelium, however limited, either in tissue culture [165] or under various experimental conditions not necessarily involving phagocytosis of fat [171, 294]. Of interest and perhaps significance are the reports that, under special circumstances, endothelium may be 'activated' to become phagocytic [51], and that such 'activation' may be observed in a variety of conditions, e.g., after histamine stimulation [28], in vascular tumors (sclerosing hemangiomas) [96], etc. DUFF *et al.* [58] have shown that colloidal thorium dioxide accumulated in the endothelium of aortic atherosclerotic lesions in the rabbits, whereas the endothelium of normal aorta does not take it up.

Nevertheless, the mere presence of fat in the endothelial cells is not synonymous with the transformation of these cells to foam cells, nor can it be considered as evidence in support of the derivation of intimal foam cells from fat-containing (lining) endothelial cells. It is surprising to find that the work of some earlier investigators has been misquoted in this respect. For example, VERSÉ [281] is quoted among authors who allegedly described the transformation of endothelial cells into foam cells [6, p. 109]. In the short abstract referred to in the above monograph, VERSÉ reported that in hypercholesterolemic rabbits, the aortic endothelium was free of fat and fat-containing endothelial cells were observed only in smaller caliber arteries, but spoke of no transformation to foam cells. However, some investigators believed in the endothelial origin of intimal foam cells. WACKER and HUECK [286] reported in 1913 the presence of cholesterol-filled intimal cells interpreted by them as endothelial cells, in the arteries of hypercholesterolemic rabbits;

SCHÖNHEIMER [246] believed that the foam cells he found in venous lesions in experimental atherosclerosis in rabbits, as well as those observed in the pulmonary vein of a nephrotic hyperlipidemic youth (as reported by BENDA), were of endothelial origin. PALLASKE [212] studied spontaneous atherosclerotic lesions in two old parrots and reported that in some types of lesions, there was evidence of endothelial transformation to foam cells; he observed similar fat-containing cells detached from the endothelial lining and believed that these were shed into the lumen. KUNTZ and SULKIN [155] studied the evolution of atherosclerotic lesions in hypercholesterolemic rabbits and, in support of their belief that foam cells were of endothelial origin, argued: 'If all the foam cells arise locally, those in the lesions of smaller arteries must be derived solely from the endothelium, for in these vessels the intima includes no other cellular elements.'

The most ardent supporter of the endothelial derivation of intimal foam cells was ALTSCHUL. He believed he was able to trace step by step the gradual transformation of fat-containing endothelial cells to intimal foam cells [4, 6]. In addition, he advocated the idea that endothelial cells proliferate in atherosclerosis and undergo metaplasia, giving rise to intimal 'intermediate' cells (see next section) that in turn may accumulate fat [5, 6]. Nevertheless, ALTSCHUL stated at the time of his last writing, that neither HUEPER [131, 132] nor he excluded the possibility (or probability?) that other cell types may become typical foam cells [6, p. 110] and that the intimal foam cells derived from the endothelium (may) join foam cells of other origin, e.g., the phagocytic mesenchymal cell of endothelial origin, immigrated monocytes or phagocytes originating from the subendothelial undifferentiated 'reserve' which, however, may have developed originally from endothelium [6, p. 103]. He concluded his deliberations on the identity and derivation of the intimal foam cells in 1954 by stating: 'Much post-mortem material will have to be examined from this point of view before any definite statement regarding human arteriosclerosis can be made' [6, p. 112].

Strong opposition to the view that endothelial cells may be the source of intimal foam cells was voiced by the authorities of the early era of atherosclerosis. KLOTZ who acknowledged that the lining endothelial cells may show deposits of fine or coarsely granular fat in their substance [151] and the foam cells were lutein-like or endothelium-like, denied that these could have an association with the lining endothelium of the blood vessels [150]. ANITSCHKOW [8] expressed the opinion that endothelial cells could not be the source of the intimal lipoid cells, because the endothelium formed throughout the entire process and in all stages of atherosclerotic lesions a single and simple layer of flat cells devoided of lipid droplets, and no transitional forms between endothelial cells and the intimal lipoid phagocytes were apparent. In the same vein, one can quote tissue culture work negating the ability of vascular endothelium to convert to (or produce) wandering cells, or to be capable of phagocytosis [179, 256]; thus, vascular endothelium must be distinguished from the reticuloendothelial cells of other organs [179, 256].

It is perhaps fair to summarize this subsection by stating that the concept of transformation of endothelial cells into foam cells, which, in turn, 'migrate' into the intima to either represent, in this location, the only foam cells or join those of other derivation, has not been established as a fact; this concept does not have the support of most contemporary investigators in the field. Whether or not the endothelial cells may become indirectly intimal cells that in the course of the process change to foam cells, is another matter, and will be dealt with elsewhere in this monograph.

Other Local Intimal Cells (Fibroblasts, Mesenchymal Cells, Smooth Muscle Cells)

Until recently, only in scattered reports reference was made to other, largely intimal connective tissue cells as being those in which lipids accumulate either exclusively or in addition to cells derived from other sources. Wacker and Hueck [286], while considering the endothelium as the source of foam cells, stated that they cannot exclude the possibility that they represent fat-filled fibroblasts. In the more advanced lesions, Klotz [150] observed that fat could be demonstrated in some of the connective tissue cells, forming wedges of deposit at the ends of the nuclei. These fatty deposits in the connective tissue cells were observed in addition to the presence of fat in cells apparently foreign to the intima, the large lutein-like cells [150, 151]. An accurate and detailed description of fat-containing cells in experimental atherosclerotic lesions in rabbits was given by Bailey in 1916 [14]. In the early lesions produced by cholesterol feeding, the intimal thickening consisted of fat-containing cells. In addition to being present in large, swollen, round or somewhat irregular cells, the fat (doubly refractile) was observed in spindle cells, a few droplets appearing at either end of the nucleus. He contended that the large fat-containing cells were reminiscent of cells present in the reticuloendothelial system and by analogy could be considered to be of endothelial type (histiocytes of Kiyono), but believed that in the intimal lesions of the aorta fibroblasts also take some part in the absorption (?) of the fat. Moreover, it seemed possible to BAILEY to follow gradations from the spindle cells (fibroblasts) with a few fat droplets to the large cells filled with fat. Lipid droplets were also observed in 'intimal connective tissue cells' in the nodular type of spontaneous lesions in parrots [212]. LEARY [160, 161] observed fat in cells which had the appearance of fibroblasts in addition to the foam cells invading from the lumen; he believed that cholesterol esters of the foam cells were broken down and cholesterol dissolved in the fibroblasts [161]. MOON and RINEHART [188] studied coronary arteries from 250 people of all ages dying suddenly of trauma or natural causes and observed that in early lesions, intracellular fat droplets were present only in intimal elongated cells (considered by them to be fibroblasts); macrophages containing lipid were almost never observed in early lesions. In the 'far advanced' lesions, lipid-filled macrophages were encountered frequently [188]. In more recent years, LAITINEN [158], UOTILA *et al.* [278], and HASS *et al.* [102] stated that in their experience, the intimal fat-containing cells were largely fibroblasts; the last group of investigators considered that the foam cells are, in addition, derived from both endothelium and macrophages [102].

In 1935, DUFF [55], one of the outstanding investigators and an acknowledged authority in the field of atherosclerosis, wrote in his extensive review on experimental cholesterol arteriosclerosis that (in addition to being present in macrophages) fatty granules were observed in the cytoplasm of spindle-shaped cells in the intimal lesions. These spindle-shaped or stellate cells found in the interstices between the (typical) foam cells were morphologically indistinguishable from fibroblasts, and were identified by him as such. DUFF then proceeded: 'The description by some of the earlier investigators of smooth muscle cells in the intima seems surely to have been due to a mistake in the identification of the spindle-shaped cells or in the recognition of the limits of the media after the internal elastic lamina has disintegrated' [55, pp. 43, 191]. This opinion, expressed by a man of great authority, may explain why, for several years to come, no reference was made to the possibility that the cells in the lesions were smooth muscle, that they may indeed be fat-containing.

Search through the older literature discloses that a few investigators indeed, observed in the intima the presence of cells they hesitated to accept as fibroblasts or endothelial derivatives. As early as in 1866, LANGHANS [159] observed in his aortic preparations the presence of peculiar intimal cells that had nothing in common with the endothelial cells and did not have the features of fibroblasts. They often appeared star-like in shape, had interconnecting cellular processes, and showed fatty metamorphosis. DOERR [54] credits VON ROKITANSKY and VIRCHOW with similar observations, but authors of the past century and the early era of this century, referred to these cells as 'Langhans' cells' when elaborating on detailed morphology, occurrence and possible functional significance of these intimal cells [153, 174]. Later, BENNINGHOFF [22], when examining human arteries, found foamy cytoplasm in intimal cells that were unusual in that they had features intermediate between fibroblasts and smooth muscle cells, and he referred to this cell type as 'Faserzelle' (translated literally it means a fiber-associated or a fiber-producing cell and may thus also include fibrocytes). By naming it distinctly 'Faserzelle' rather than 'Fibrocyte', he emphasized that these were two different cells. BENNINGHOFF [22] described the cell as having a well-defined cellular contour with star-like extension and a cytoplasm of 'low density' in which fibrillae (particularly in cytoplasmic extensions) could be identified. The cells were particularly well stained with the iron hematoxylin stain. They could 'turn' into macrophages and cholesterol ester-containing phagocytes. He referred to the fact that prior to his observations, similar cells were reported by FLEMMING and later by LANGHANS [159] in the aortic intima. However, BENNINGHOFF [22], although recognizing that some features of these cells were those of smooth muscle cells, did not actually state that they represent the latter.

As far as it can be determined, the first author who stated that in atherosclerotic lesions fat is present in intimal smooth muscle cells was JORES. According to KLOTZ[1] [150, pp. 423–424], JORES had noticed that a mixed type of hyperplasia of the musculo-elastic layer with fatty degeneration and superimposed 'regeneration' (? proliferation) of connective tissue could be observed in lesions. JORES had restricted the term arteriosclerosis to intimal changes characterized by hyperplasia of the musculo-elastic layer, splitting of the internal elastic lamina and accompanying fatty degeneration of the longitudinal muscle fibers. Moreover, he considered the fatty degeneration in the (superimposed) connective tissue thickening to be secondary to degenerative processes in the deep musculo-elastic layer. Whereas it is not certain from the above whether the smooth muscle cells containing fat represented, indeed, always cells of the musculo-elastic layer, or were mistaken by

[1] Regretfully, the references to JORES' work given by KLOTZ in his publications [150, 151] were either incorrectly quoted by him (Zieglers Beiträge *13:* 726, 1902; Zbl. allg. Path. path. Anat. *14:* 865, 869, 1903) in reference to the citation relevant to the smooth muscle cells, incomplete (Arteriosklerose, Bonn 1903), or inaccessible to us (Wesen und Entwicklung der Arteriosklerose, Bergmann, Wiesbaden 1903).

JORES as belonging to this layer, the fact remains that he observed fatty degeneration of intimal smooth muscle cells in atherosclerotic lesions. KLOTZ' [150, 151] own observations were largely in agreement with those of JORES, and he concluded among others that... 'Deep areas of degeneration also show the involvement of the muscle cells of the intima.' [150, p. 429]. Nevertheless, KLOTZ reported that he had observed repeatedly proliferative changes in the superficial connective tissue without involvement of the musculo-elastic layer, in which the newly developed tissue showed fatty deposits in the connective tissue cells, as well as the presence of cells apparently foreign to the intima, i.e., the large lutein-like cells, which were loaded with fat. However, he did not characterize further the fat-containing, 'connective tissue cells' in the newly developing connective tissue.

Further reference to the presence of fat in smooth muscle cells in the lesions was made by PALLASKE in 1930 in the aforementioned publication on the spontaneous atherosclerotic lesions in parrots [212, p. 68]. Thus (in addition to the foam cells he believed to be derived from endothelium and fat found in connective tissue cells), lipid was observed in the intimal smooth muscle cells, and in severe lesions, also in the medial smooth muscle cells. Accumulation of fat in the latter apparently resulted in cellular disintegration.

Little more was said in the literature on the subject of fat-containing smooth muscle or similar cells until 1944, when ALTSCHUL [4] reported the results of his histological examination of atherosclerotic lesions in a basilar artery. In addition to finding foam cells he believed to be derived from the endothelium, he observed under the endothelial lining connective tissue cells with features distinguishing them from fibroblasts. They were star-shaped and had numerous fibrillar processes. ALTSCHUL did not regard these to be related to, or identical with the reticular cells or mesenchymal cells, but believed he was able to trace these to gradually transforming endothelial cells, just as, according to him, the foam cells were derived from endothelial cells. He maintained that the change in appearance which occurs when endothelial cells become displaced into the subendothelial layer and lose their function, i.e., to line blood vessels, might be regarded as a regression or dedifferentiation, and the fatty metamorphosis of these (former) endothelial cells as degeneration. He thus asserted that both forms of intimal foam cells were derived from endothelium. Even though his attention was drawn to these unusual cells at that time, it was not until some six years later that he formulated his opinion clearer regarding the nature of these cells on the one hand, and on the other actually described the appearance of cytoplasmic vacuoles in these; he was convinced that the vacuoles represented fat lost in tissue processing [5]. In addition to these cells originating from the endothelium via dedifferentiation (or metaplasia), ALTSCHUL believed that similar cells may be derived from the medial smooth muscle cells that migrate into the intima in experimental arteriosclerosis and in hyperplastic type of human arteriosclerosis [5, p. 54]; the latter observation was thus in accord with that of JORES made half a century earlier. ALTSCHUL contended that the presence of smooth muscle cells 'in the intima in human atherosclerosis had been overlooked or not recorded because judged most improbable' – no doubt a reference to the above-quoted statement by DUFF [55]. He acknowledged that the intimal cells under consideration were identical with BENNINGHOFF'S 'Faserzellen' and the cells of LANGHANS, but: 'I suggested changing BENNINGHOFF'S term "transitional cells" or "Faserzellen" to "intermediate cells" because it is not established that the Langhans cells, if not arrested by death, would have continued their metamorphosis towards either muscle cells or fibroblasts' [6, p. 43]. But in another passage of his writing he states: 'In experimental cholesterol arteriosclerosis the intermediate cell type may also be found, but usually dedifferentiation has either not gone far enough and one is able to recognize the source of these cells – endothelium or smooth muscle – or it has apparently already gone beyond the intermediate state, in which case the cells are transformed into fibroblasts. These observations coincide with those made on the dedifferentiation of endothelium in general' [5, p. 65].

Without wishing to minimize the role ALTSCHUL played in drawing our attention to the presence of the cells in atherosclerotic lesions we now agree are smooth muscle cells, one must admit that his writings, largely published in the form of two monographs [5, 6], are extremely difficult to read and comprehend. Through the generosity of the late Dr. ALTSCHUL, one of the present writers has been in the possession of both monographs for many years and, despite the familiarity with his work, finds it extremely difficult to gather the information reflecting Dr. ALTSCHUL'S views, as they are scattered throughout the often repetitious or contradictory monographs (see above), and one has the impression that his thoughts were seldom 'thought out to the end'. Perhaps it is for these reasons that his statements and observations are often misquoted in the literature on the one hand, and on the other, shying reading the difficult communications, people assume that 'having said one thing he must have also said all there was to be said', and ascribe to him work he did not do and statements he never made. Summarizing ALTSCHUL'S contribution to the present state of knowledge regarding the cells under consideration, one may state that by being the first in modern times to write in English on the subject, he drew the attention of the North American investigators to the presence of these intimal cells in atherosclerotic lesions. However, these cells were described at least as early as 1866 by LANGHANS [159], considered by BENNINGHOFF [22] as transitional forms between smooth muscle cells and fibroblasts, and recognized to be smooth muscle cells by JORES at the turn of the century. The presence of fat in these cells in atherosclerotic lesions was also recorded by the above and other investigators prior to ALTSCHUL. Nevertheless, ALTSCHUL compiled (although in a rather confusing form) much of the information pertaining to the subject (until the middle of this century) and therein, too, lies his achievement.

It was not until 1960 that fat-containing smooth muscle cells were unequivocally identified in the fatty streaks of experimental [214] and human [74] atherosclerosis with the help of the electron microscope. PARKER identified these cells in the coronary arteries of hypercholesterolemic rabbits [214], whereas GEER *et al.* [74] observed similar cells in human aortic atherosclerotic lesions. The latter observations were extended [75, 111] and the fact established that in one form of early atherosclerotic lesions (fatty dots and streaks), lipid accumulates in the smooth muscle cells and later in cells that appear to be macrophages. Foam cells result from the accumulation of large amounts of fat in both types of cells. When derived from the smooth muscle cells, the fat-filled cells are referred to as myogenic foam cells [15]. With these facts established, the inquiry into the nature, etiology and pathogenesis of atherosclerosis entered a new era.

Before leaving the subject of the nature of fat-containing cells in atherosclerotic lesions, it appears desirable to review also this matter, as it pertains to fat-containing cells in arterial mural thrombi, largely because mural thrombosis has been acknowledged by some to represent one form of the early atherosclerotic lesions, and most investigators agree that it represents one of the important mechanisms by which the lesions may grow. There is not much information in the literature available on this matter; most pertains to the experimental embolization of the pulmonary tree by various means and to subsequent organization of the emboli – all efforts to test the hypothesis of VON ROKITANSKY that organization of mural thrombi give rise to (some) lesions of atherosclerosis. In 1948, HARRISON [100] found lipid only in one of the lesions produced in the pulmonary arteries of rabbits by the injection of finely fragmented human blood clot; the lesions were otherwise indistinguishable from spontaneous atherosclerosis. To test whether the nature of the introduced emboli have any bearing upon the morphology of these pulmonary lesions, HEPTINSTALL [125] injected clots from hypercholesterolemic blood of rabbits to a group of rabbits on normal diet and to another group fed a cholesterol-containing diet. Large numbers of fat-containing cells were observed in the intima of the pulmonary arteries of rabbits of the latter group, whereas only few were present in the former. HEPTINSTALL referred to these cells as 'cholesterol-containing macrophages' or foam cells (interchangeably) and, whereas he discussed the various possible mechanisms by which these cells may accumulate, he did not consider that these cells may be anything else but macrophages, with the following exception: 'The proliferation of endothelial cells may also play *some* part by taking on the role of phagocytes for cholesterol' [125, p. 444]. In final analysis, HEPTINSTALL believed that the most likely explanation of the increased 'deposition' of fat-containing macrophages in the intima of embolized arteries was a consequence of an intense initial arteritis following injection of emboli. He believed that at the time of acute arteritis there was migration of foam cells into the intima due to increased permeability, and that these cells remained in the area after resolution had occurred.

The lipid-containing cells that appeared in the course of organization of emboli from thrombi used in the experiments of CHANDLER and HAND [36, 98] were also considered to be macrophages. However, the authors believed that the presence of lipid in the macrophages resulted from ingestion of platelets by these cells. These authors were the first investigators to demonstrate that lipid-containing arterial lesions may develop in animals without dietary lipid manipulation.

In human atherosclerotic lesions, scattered macrophages were observed in unorganized aortic mural thrombi [192]. These were closely applied to the clumps and bands of fibrin remnants, and some cells had the typical appearance of lipophages. The latter increased in number in advanced lesions and often accumulated at the base of entirely unorganized thrombi which in turn were covered by layers of recent thrombi. These lipophages distintegrated in advanced lesions providing a nidus for atheroma formation. The mechanisms of lipid accumulation in these cells were not discussed, nor was consideration given to the possibility that the lipophages may be derived from cells other than macrophages [192].

This area, i.e., the identification of cells containing fat under these and similar thrombotic conditions as they relate to the process of atherosclerosis, requires further exploration and should provide a fruitful field for research, as it is quite logical to assume at present that some, if not most, of these cells are smooth muscle cells rather than macrophages.

Cells Associated with Connective Tissue Proliferation

The first detailed account of the morphology of atherosclerotic lesions in man was provided by VIRCHOW [283, 283], and even if we today do not agree necessarily with the sequence of events taking place in tissues as proposed by him, his description remains amazingly accurate. VIRCHOW was impressed with an almost neoplastic proliferation of connective tissue of the intima in the stage of 'irritation' in atherosclerosis, and in describing the formation of the sclerotic plaque considered that this process was initiated by enlargement and multiplication of cells generally designated by him as connective tissue cells (Bindegewebskörperchen = fibroblasts). He observed that fat droplets accumulated in these cells which '. . . often were star-shaped and had anastomozing processes.'

Thereafter, LANGHANS[2] [159] concerning himself with the morphology and histogenesis of atherosclerotic lesions of human arteries, recorded his observations that differ little from our present-day knowledge. He described among others focal intimal lesions consisting of 'transparent' gelatinous elevations containing cells that were either star-like in shape or round, and pointed out that in the aorta, these were located in the superficial rather than deep parts of the intima and thus, could not represent 'hypertrophy' of the elements in the depth of the intima, as proposed by some of his predecessors. This change represented also the basis for the occurrence of the grossly visible cartilage-like plates (white plaques). Microscopic examination of these plaques revealed that they often consisted of two or even several distinct 'subdivisions', i.e., layers which were distinguishable from each other by the state of maturation, direction and number of both cellular elements and connective tissue fibers. These layers seemed to be 'added' to the lesion from the luminal aspect and stretched out (thinned) laterally to blend with the surrounding (normal) intima. Of particular interest to him was the appearance and 'behaviour' of cells in these layers; he found these to be either star-like or round, and observed unequivocal evidence of mitoses in the latter. The round cells had the tendency to appear in small groups, at the lines of demarcation between the individual layers, and although often found in the interstices of the interconnecting processes of the star-like cells, they were observed also in the absence of the latter. Indeed, LANGHANS believed that he could observe various stages of transformation between the round and

[2] It is of some curiosity that LANGHANS' name was misspelled in his own original publication and reads: Langhaas instead of Langhans.

the star-like cell. Thus, the nucleus of the former elongated and enlarged, and the cytoplasm acquired a considerable size and several long processes which seemed interconnecting with, or abutting on similar extensions from neighboring cells. He observed again unequivocal mitoses of these star-like cells and arrived at the conclusion that division of the latter gives rise to either identical cells, or to the round cells. Thus, each of the two types (morphological forms) could give rise, or transform to the other. Moreover, he maintained that in the normal intima only the star-like cells are present and when the pathological process sets in, these cells multiply giving rise also to the round cells. Furthermore, he speculated that this ability to transform from one form of a cell to another may be a property common to all proliferating tissues of man and in analogy with those observed by von Recklinghausen in the cornea of a frog. He ventured also to express the opinion that in all probability the star-like cells are *contractile* and are capable of migration, although admitting that the latter property would have to be substantiated. Concerning the morphological features of the star-like cells in atherosclerotic lesions, he observed that these differed somewhat from those of similar cells in the normal intima: The nucleus was longer but narrower, the cells were considerably larger as was also the width of the cellular processes; in the extensions of these cellular processes, bundles of fine fibrils could be observed.

The relation of the elongated processes to those of neighboring cells on the one hand and to the extracellular substances on the other, could be best visualized by silver impregnation techniques; the extracellular substance resembled islets surrounded by an extensive system of canals consisting of a net of intercommunicating cell processes, and it was often impossible to determine where the boundary of one cell began and the other ended. The arrangement and direction of the cell bodies and their processes changed in lesions consisting of layers: Whereas in the most superficial layer the cells and their processes were parallel to the endothelial surface, the cells either assumed a direction tangential to the lumen or their processes extended perpendicularly toward the superficial as well as deeper layers in the interior of the lesion. No special reference was made to the possible relation of these cells to the extracellular substances, although by implication it may be assumed that, with one exception, these cells are responsible for the elaboration of these substances; exception was made explicitly by Langhans with respect to the formation of elastic tissue in lesions. He maintained that lesions of large arteries show paucity of elastic fibers, whereas those in smaller arteries abound in these. The elastic fibers, when present, may be the result of either splitting of the existing elastic elements or represent new formation, but the latter is *not* the product of the cells ('... die Neubildung ... ist nicht aus Zellen hervorgegangen.' [159, p. 208]. The intercellular substances resemble those of normal intima and the fibers are parallel to the endothelial surface. Often there is a gelatinous change evident, but he could not confirm the presence of mucin in such areas; rather, he observed alterations in fibrillarity on the one hand and, on the other, a considerable increase in the homogeneous ground substance, particularly in the superficial layers of the lesion. LANGHANS then proceeds to describe the presence of fat in the lesions in the course of what he considered to be the morphogenetic steps in the development of the full-blown fat-containing atherosclerotic lesions and taking issues on many aspects of the pathogenesis and morphology with VIRCHOW – all matters of importance, but outside the realm of this subsection.

The work of LANGHANS has been reviewed purposely in some detail for several reasons. It is most astonishing to learn that almost a century ago, LANGHANS not only described the cells in proliferating connective tissue of atherosclerotic lesions with great accuracy, but stated in addition that these cells were the same as those populating the normal intima (with definable alterations), were probably contractile and mobile, divided visibly and in so doing gave rise to a 'round' cell that in turn divided and transformed to the typical star-shaped cell under consideration; the 'round' cell no doubt corresponds to the immature precursor of the smooth muscle cell found in addition to the latter by electron microscopy in proliferating atherosclerotic lesions. Why, then, did we have to 'rediscover' all these observations of monumental work and original thoughts of LANGHANS and it took us almost one hundred years to do so? There are two possible interrelated reasons that may be responsible for the almost complete oblivion of his work. LANGHANS had the courage of conviction to contradict and question the teachings of VIRCHOW, the giant in science of his era, particularly on the subject of the morphogenesis of atherosclerotic lesions. Instead of disregarding only the issues at contention and accepting the validity of his morphological observations and thoughts, the pathologists of these and following years simply ignored all of his work with only a few notable exceptions that have not 'survived' to modern times. Interrelated with the above has been the problem of failure (for whatever reason) of the English-speaking scientific community to review in detail work written in German. Before leaving the subject of LANGHANS' contributions, it should be emphasized that he did not refer to the cells in question as smooth muscle cells.

Around the turn of the century, JORES (quoted by KLOTZ [149, pp. 715–716]) classified the focal progressive intimal changes as being either hyperplastic or regenerative. According to him, the hyperplastic thickening, consisting largely of focal excessive development of the musculo-elastic layer, was the result of a 'hyper-physiological' process. Factors that throw an increased strain upon this intimal muscle layer lead to the hypertrophy, and when the strain is persisting or severe, degeneration takes place in the muscle cells of this layer. On the other hand, the regenerative lesions were superficial to the musculo-elastic layer and developed independent of any changes of this layer. This regenerative process, regarded by JORES as a connective tissue proliferation of inflammatory nature, lacked the features of inflammation observed in other tissues, and the lesions were considered to result from the proliferation of the 'superficial cells'. Only a single type of cell was observed in early stages of development and was considered by some to be of endothelial, by others of connective tissue origin. Fine elastic fibrils appeared later in the development of this type of intimal plaque [149]. Several years later, when KLOTZ examined microscopically the focal intimal elevations of the human aorta around the orifices of the intercostal arteries, he, too, considered these to be the outcome of an inflammatory process accompanied by progressive (as well as degenerative) changes of the intima. Accordingly, repair was accomplished by proliferation of the connective tissues of the inner intimal layer and showed some hyperplasia of the musculo-elastic layer. He classified this process as arteriosclerosis (= atherosclerosis). In the early stages of the process, he observed in the intima stellate connective tissue cells which were best appreciated in sections cut 'on the flat'. These cells formed a meshwork with fairly wide spaces, 'looking not unlike the fibrous tissue cells of cultures *in vitro*. The wandering (?) cells are most frequently found near the surface while few are seen, in the early stages, at the inner border of the media.'[3]

KLOTZ made no further reference to these cells. In final analysis, JORES and his followers (e.g., KLOTZ) observed hyperplasia of smooth muscle cells in what was considered one form of atherosclerosis, insisting that these cells are involved only in the process localized to the musculo-elastic layer in the

[3] KLOTZ [150] quotes among others in this connection the work of BURROWS [33] on the cultivation of tissues of the chick embryo. On reviewing this publication, no reference to stellate connective tissue cells described by KLOTZ was found, and the only mention of cells is as follows: 'The most actively growing element in the preparations is the interstitial connective tissue cell. These cells begin to spread into the plasma either as single cells or a layer of cells...'

depth of the intima and considered that an entirely different cell type appeared in the other, i.e., regenerative type of atherosclerosis localized in the superficial intima. No systematized attempt was made to elaborate on the relation of the proliferating extracellular substances to the cells in either location.

Renewed stimulus for further examination and identification of cells associated with proliferative aspects of atherosclerotic lesions was provided by the experimental hypercholesterolemic intimal lesions in rabbits, and the numerous variations and permutations in design and species employed that followed. ANITSCHKOW [7] himself observed even in the early lesions produced experimentally in hypercholesterolemic rabbits, growing numbers of stationary elongated cells in the subendothelial layers; they were situated between the large macrophagic foam cells, and coincided with the proliferation of elastic and argyrophilic fibers in the subendothelial layer. As the lesions advanced, collagen fibers also appeared and single elongated cells with oval nuclei could be seen between the fibers. In regressive stages of the lesions (1.5–2 years after cessation of cholesterol feeding), cells that ANITSCHKOW was now willing to define as fibroblasts, were present in the focal intimal thickening which remained after the reabsorption of lipids. In his experimental series, BAILEY [14] observed that, as the lesions progressed, there was a marked proliferation of fibroblasts and an abundant formation of collagen and fine elastic fibers especially in the upper (luminal) portion of the lesion. He also observed that by even slight modifications of the experiments, the degree of fibrosis could be altered, a fact re-emphasized again in modern times [293]. In lesions of young persons, LEARY [160] observed fibroblastic tissue produced in the subendothelial areas with young fibroblasts 'engulfing and metabolizing' the lipid that gradually disappeared from the lesions. Repair with only minimal scarring followed, since – according to him – the young fibroblastic tissue does not form collagen. LEARY refers to the cells present as fibrolipophages, and it is probable that the lesions under consideration were advanced fatty streaks rather than largely connective tissue lesions.

In his detailed account on experimental cholesterol atherosclerosis, DUFF reported that with progression of lesions '... fibroblasts come into prominence. They proliferate extensively in the deeper layers of the intimal thickening and frequently form a compact fibrous layer just beneath the intimal[4] surface. There is a marked increase in fibroglia and elastic fibrils, the latter

[4] We feel that the late Professor DUFF meant endothelial rather than intimal surface.

often showing a connection with the splitting internal elastic lamina' [55, p. 94]. Since the relatively frequent occurrence of mitotic figures in the stellate fibroblastic cells (as well as in the globular foam cells) in aortic lesions induced in hypercholesterolemic rabbits seemed to have been overlooked by previous workers in experimental atherosclerosis, he set out to investigate this phenomenon with McMillan [182]. On the basis of their morphological assessment of incidence and phase of the mitotic figures encountered in a single section of the entire length of the aorta, they concluded that mitotic figures were observed in all layers of lesions, but were most frequent in the more superficial cells, and that: 'Regardless of what theory is proposed relative to the derivation and original source of the foam cells and fibroblasts in the lesions of experimental cholesterol atherosclerosis, it is apparent that a considerable proportion of them arise *in situ* by mitotic division' [182, p 182]. Thus, the observation of Langhans regarding the mitotic division in human atherosclerotic lesions was also applicable to experimental lesions, but at the same time, the idea that the cells associated with the connective tissue proliferation were anything else but fibroblasts became firmly entrenched. This applied also to observations in man. On the basis of their morphological examination of human coronary arteries in a large series of hearts, Moon and Rinehart [188] concluded that, of the various stages in the development of lesions, subendothelial proliferation of fibroblasts was the earliest phenomenon. This was seen in the intima of all individuals over twenty years of age; in most of the early lesions, fibroblasts were dispersed in mucoid ground substance. Moreover, there was a remarkably close association of fibroblastic proliferation and degeneration of elastic tissue in the earliest sclerotic changes of coronary arteries; the second stage of development was characterized by maturation of collagen fibers and regeneration of elastic fibers.

Finally, the domain of fibroblasts in human atherosclerosis was enlarged in 1952, when Crawford and Levene [43] set out to test the validity of Duguid's revival of the thrombogenic (or encrustation) theory of von Rokitansky. Indeed, they found surface depositions on the human aortic intima and, in tracing the various stages from fresh mural thrombosis to complete organization, observed that, from the luminal aspect, the latter usually proceeded in the absence of capillaries and that the cells responsible for the organization of the superficial part of the thrombus were fibroblasts.

In 1955, a team of Canadian pathologists began morphological investigations into the nature of fibrogenesis in atherosclerotic lesions of man, utilizing aortae and coronary arteries obtained at necropsies. In the course of these studies, it was noticed that whenever a lesion represented what was interpreted as steps in the organization of exogenous (to the intima) proteins (i.e., in the gelatinous elevations and in mural thrombi), there were large numbers of cells with features that could not be fitted easily into any category of standard orthodox teaching. Review of the writings of the contemporary authors (as quoted above) yielded the information that these cells were fibroblasts – a concept unacceptable to the team. Totally unaware at that time of the writings of LANGHANS and ALTSCHUL, they concluded on the basis of their histochemical studies that these cells were smooth muscle cells and presented their preliminary results in 1956 [104] before the American Society for the Study of Arteriosclerosis (now: Council on Arteriosclerosis of the American Heart Association). This unheard of heretical view[5] was vehemently rejected by all present with the notable exception of the late Dr. ALTSCHUL (who subsequently donated his two monographs [5, 6] to one of the present authors and a member of that team) and Dr. J. F. A. (Joe) MCMANUS, the then Professor of Pathology at the University of Alabama Medical Center, Birmingham, Ala. Contentious was not only the proposed presence of smooth muscle cells in the lesions, but the view that these cells were responsible for the organization and thus for connective tissue elaboration, a property substantiated by the same group later on the basis of their histochemical work [106–109, 112, 191]. The cells that were concerned with the organization of superficial layers of mural thrombi, and the serous or serofibrinous insudate in the gray gelatinous intimal elevations, were also observed to populate the white or pearly-white atherosclerotic plaques. They were elongated, parallel to the surface and arranged in the longitudinal axis of the arteries; the slender slightly acidophilic cytoplasm with many tapering processes contained deeply acidophilic and PTAH-positive myofibrils arranged parallel to the long axis. The coarser of the myofibrils appeared to extend beyond the cellular boundary and 'communicate' with similar fibrils of the neighboring cells, and interlacing with each other. The nucleus was elongated, cigar-like in shape and had blunt ends. The cells were often seen in a stage of apparent contraction; the nucleus assumed then a 'snake-fence' appearance, the cytoplasm was broadened in the perinuclear area and its poles with the extending myofibrils were 'pulled' towards the center of the

[5] An abstract on this subject submitted for presentation at the Annual Meeting of the American Association of Pathologists and Bacteriologists in 1957 was rejected (probably considered as nonsense) and read only by title [106]; it was, however, accepted for presentation at the Annual Meeting of the Federation of American Societies for Experimental Biology the following year [107].

cell. A striking phenomenon was the intimate association of these cells with formed connective tissue elements and in very young connective tissue area abounding in acid mucopolysaccharides-rich ground substance, the connective tissue fibers appeared first in close vicinity (or contact) with the cellular boundary. This applied to the developing elastic and collagen fibers and to delicate silver-positive reticulin fibrils. Moreover, a prominent layer of PAS-positive substance that was not collagen was closely applied to the cell body. Subsequently, it became apparent on electron microscopic examination that this PAS-positive substance represents the basement membrane of the smooth muscle cells. Since no other cells were observed in the human lesions examined, it was concluded that these smooth muscle cells were entirely responsible for connective tissue elaboration. FLOREY *et al.* [68] supported the above concepts on the basis of their examination of the pseudointima that lined fabric aortic grafts in baboon, and they were firmly established for human lesions on the basis of electron microscopy [116, 119].

There is nothing inherently unusual in the observation that smooth muscle cells elaborate connective tissue elements in atherosclerotic lesions, as it had been a well-established fact that they have a similar function in other organs (e.g., uterus) and in the developmental stages of arteries.

Unifying Concepts and Summary

It may be stated in conclusion that in the sixth decade of this century, it became firmly established that the smooth muscle cell is the principal cell involved in both regressive and progressive changes taking place in the process of atherosclerosis, both in man and in experimental animals. The regressive changes consist of fatty metamorphosis and, in progressive lesions, this cell proliferates organizing exogenous proteins and elaborating connective tissue elements. Most of the above features, as they refer to the identity of this cell, were observed sporadically in the past (even in the last century), but it was truly left to the investigators of modern times to establish that this cell is a common denominator playing a role in the development of all types of atherosclerotic lesions. Whether or not this is also true for the inception of these lesions remains to be tested next, and presents a challenge for future investigators.

III. Arterial Structure and Reaction to Injury

General Considerations of Architecture

The systemic arterial vasculature begins at the aortic valve ring of the heart and courses to all tissues of the body with conduits of progressively decreasing lumen diameter and wall thickness. Arteries are classified as elastic, muscular, and arterioles. Muscular arteries are further subdivided as large, medium, or small. Unfortunately, this classification lacks rigid definition of size or structure of the various arteries; loose usage of terms, such as large artery or small artery, does not convey the same meaning to different readers. It is not within the province of this presentation to attempt clarification of this terminological problem. We refer to an artery as an elastic artery if the media of the artery is composed of laminae of smooth muscle and elastic plates. A muscular artery has a media composed predominately of smooth muscle cells and has only scattered small fibers of elastica. Endothelium and smooth muscle are the cells common to mammalian arteries of all sizes; the connective tissue components vary. Large arteries contain abundant elastic tissue. As the vessel becomes smaller and the wall correspondingly thinner, the large elastic plates of the media are replaced by small elastic fibers, and, in medium to small-size muscular arteries, there may be no elastic tissue present. The medial connective tissue skeleton of muscular arteries consists predominantly of collagen and basement membranes, and that of arterioles almost exclusively of basement membranes.

Histologically, the arterial wall has three tunics or coats. Adjacent to the arterial lumen is the innermost coat or intima. The intima includes the endothelium, tissue space beneath endothelium and the internal elastic lamina (or membrane). The media extends from the innermost or medial aspect of the internal elastic lamina to the outermost layer of smooth muscle or to elastic fibers comprising an external elastic membrane. The adventitial coat begins at the outer limit of the media and gradually blends with the surrounding tissue.

Intima

The only cell type found consistently in the intima of a normal artery at birth is endothelium. With growth and maturation, smooth muscle cells may appear in the intima between the endothelium and the internal elastic lamina. Whether the appearance of smooth muscle cells in the intima can be considered normal or abnormal is a matter of definition of normal. Diffuse intimal thickening containing smooth muscle and perhaps other cells will be considered in chapter IV. A normal artery obtained at birth and examined by light microscopy usually shows the endothelium resting upon the internal elastic lamina with scant intervening connective tissue elements or apparent tissue space. There are variations in the appearance of the internal elastic lamina of large arteries. The thoracic aorta in most species has an internal elastic lamina composed of a closely packed network of small elastic fibers. The abdominal segment of the aorta and muscular arteries have an internal elastic membrane which is a thick fenestrated elastic plate. With aging and intimal thickening, the internal elastic membrane may disappear in some species and be replaced by a network of small elastic fibers [146]. This change in the appearance of the internal elastic membrane is often referred to as 'fraying' of the internal elastic membrane. The term 'fraying' may not be strictly correct. We are not sure whether this change in appearance represents fraying; it may be that the membrane has been resorbed and the network of small elastic fibers seen is newly formed.

Media

The architecture of the media distinguishes an elastic artery from a muscular one. Layers or laminae of smooth muscle sandwiched between two elastic plates and tissue space containing collagen constitute the basic structure of the elastic arterial media. Smooth muscle cells between the elastic plates are placed so that their long axis has a spiral orientation in relation to the long axis of the artery [268]. The angle of the spiral varies from layer to layer [218]. The angle is more acute in the inner (i.e., laminae near the intima are more nearly circumferential) than in the outer layers of the media.

The plates of elastin in the media have numerous branches which extend between the enclosed smooth muscle cells and into the connective tissue space between the laminae of elastin and smooth muscle. The size of the connective tissue space between laminae of elastin and smooth muscle varies with species and age. The connective tissue space and its collagen content increases with age. The media of mammalian arteries contains only smooth muscle cells [217–219]. Avian species have another cell type in the media in addition to smooth muscle [42, 197], the interlamellar connective tissue cell.

The media of a muscular artery is composed of closely packed smooth muscle cells, with their long axis oriented so that they form a spiral in relation to the long axis of the vessel. Thus, as the cells contract, the diameter of the lumen diminishes and the vessel shortens. Medial smooth muscle cells appear to coil in the direction of the long axis of the vessel, with the proximal and distal extremities of one cell in proximity to the next cell in a single file arrangement. As we shall see later, such a single file arrangement is an oversimplification of the structure, as by electron microscopy lateral attachments are found between smooth muscle cells in the media of muscular arteries. Collagen and small fibers of elastic tissue are present in varying amounts between the laminae of smooth muscle. Generally the larger the muscular artery the more abundant are collagen and elastic fibers between the layers of smooth muscle.

Adventitia

The adventitia of most arteries consists of a loose arrangement of collagen, elastic fibers, fibroblasts, blood vessels, lymphatics, and nerves. Adventitial structures gradually blend with the surrounding tissue, and there is no structure that externally limits the adventitia. In large elastic arteries, the adventitial vessels (vasa vasorum) extend into the media for variable distances. The studies of WOLINSKY and GLAGOV [295, 296] have clearly shown that the presence of medial vasa vasorum in mammalian elastic arteries depends on the number of elastin-smooth muscle lamellar units in the media. Arteries having more than 29 units have medial vasa vasorum and those with less than that number do not. Small animals such as the mouse, rat, cat, and rabbit have fewer than 29 lamellar units in the media and thus do not have medial vasa vasorum. Normal muscular arteries in all species do not have medial vasa vasorum. The nerve fibers in the adventitia do not penetrate into the media of either elastic or muscular arteries [213, 218, 219, 229]. The transmission of nervous impulses within the arterial media must be by a smooth muscle cell to smooth muscle cell route.

Fine Structure

Endothelium

The shape of endothelial cells has been described as being more cuboidal in elastic than in muscular arteries [197], but structures within the endothelial cells are identical in both [229]. The variation in shape that has been noted very likely reflects the degree of contraction of the artery. The typical endothelial cell is squamoid with a centrally placed nucleus. The cytoplasm, extending from the thick central portion of the cell, gradually thins. The extensions of the cell are in contact with adjacent cells forming a complete cellular pavement separating the lumen of the vessel from the underlying intima with no gaps or pores present. At intervals about the cell circumference, there are specialized cell-to-cell attachments, tight junctions or desmosomes [213]. Cell-to-cell apposition between the tight junctions is a regular space between the outer laminae of the plasma membranes measuring approximately 100–200 Å in width. The junction between two endothelial cells varies from a complex hand-in-glove arrangement of cytoplasmic processes to two thin processes barely approximating each other. The absence of a circumferential seal of the terminal bar type makes it possible for cells or fluids to pass into the arterial intima without having to pass through the endothelium [71]. An endothelial structure that corresponds to the surface coating demonstrable in light microscope preparations has been identified in electron micrographs of elastic arteries [71]; this observation awaits confirmation.

The endothelium may show cytoplasmic finger-like extensions into both the lumen and intima. The extensions into the lumen resemble microvilli; those extending into the intima possibly are an artifact produced by contraction of the vessel. The luminal and intimal endothelial plasma membrane shows multiple invaginations of the micropinocytotic type.

Cytoplasmic organelles in endothelium of normal arteries are few in number [213], compared to metabolically active cells such as liver or renal tubules. The cell contains scattered small mitochondria which generally are round in shape [229], scattered profiles of endoplasmic reticulum which are largely of the rough type, Golgi membranes in close proximity to the nucleus [197], and free ribonucleoprotein particles scattered throughout the cytoplasm. In addition, a variable number of thin filaments are present in the cytoplasm; these are typically located in the basal portion of the cell [197]. The filaments measure approximately 70 Å in diameter and have been considered to represent tonofilaments analogous to those observed in other types of epithelium. Recent electron microscopic work [169] lends support to the previously held opinion by some investigators, that the endothelial cells are contractile. Fluorescein-labelled rabbit antiserum to human platelet thrombosthenin, a contractile protein having the physicochemical characteristics of smooth muscle actomyosin [24, 206], specifically stains endothelial cells. Moreover, fluorescein-labelled antisera to human uterine actomyosin or myosin stained specifically the endothelial cells of arteries, veins and capillaries, whereas no such staining was observed when fluorescein-labelled antisera to either human cardiac muscle actomyosin or myosin or to human skeletal muscle actomyosin or myosin was employed [20]. Histochemical studies also suggested that certain endothelial cells give staining reactions similar to those of smooth muscle cells [227].

Endothelial Basement Membrane

Adjacent to the basal plasma membrane of endothelium, there is a basement membrane of varying thickness and appearance. The basement membrane is composed of a moderately electron-dense flocculent-appearing material in which thin filaments may be seen. A fine fibrillary or filamentous attachment of the basal plasma membrane of endothelium to the basement membrane has been described, with the fibrils varying from 20 to 80 Å in diameter [277]. Firm attachment of endothelium to the basement membrane has been demonstrated at focal areas; the cytoplasm is increased in electron density relative to adjacent areas [277]. These areas of attachment differ morphologically from the hemidesmosomes that have been described in other cell types. Attachment of the endothelial basement membrane to the internal elastic lamina by similar 20–80 Å fibrils also has been proposed [277].

Subendothelial Intimal Tissues

The intima of normal, young postnatal arteries usually is devoid of cells except endothelium. Intimal cells have been described in 'normal' arteries that have the morphological characteristics of smooth muscle. Between the basement membrane of the endothelium and the internal elastic lamina, there is a variable number of formed elements of connective tissue, unit fibrils of collagen, microfibrils and elastic fibers. The collagen is typical in appearance except that the diameter of the fibrils has been reported to be smaller than that seen in the adventitia [146, 148, 197]. The microfibrils vary in diameter from approximately 20 to 140 Å. Marked variation in size and diameter can be observed in a single micrograph indicating that the variation is not the result of species differences, artifacts of preparation, or grazing sections. Microfibrils similar to those described in arterial tissue have been seen in connective tissues at many other sites [115], and thus the microfibril must be a common constituent to all connective tissues. Present information is not adequate to conclude whether these microfibrils of varying diameter have the same or differing chemical composition. As will be described in the next paragraph, similar fibrils are involved in the formation of elastic fibers. It has been proposed that the microfibrils are a common structural component of both collagen and elastin [115], but this has not been proven. The suggestion that microfibrils 20–80 Å in diameter may serve to attach cells to basement membrane and basement membrane to elastic fibers, while attractive, also is not proven.

The literature on the structure of elastin is confusing due to varying methods of tissue preparation, interpretation of stains used in electron microscopy, and observations made in man and animals of varying age [93, 113, 115, 146, 158, 197, 213, 219, 238, 279]. Mature elastin appears homogeneous and in epoxy embedding media is electron-lucent. On staining with uranyl acetate or lead, elastic fibers become more electron-dense and remain homogeneous. Two structures are visible in newly forming elastic fibers [93, 113, 115]; peripheral microfibrils up to 100 Å in diameter, composed of what appears to be either end-to-end vesicles or double coiled filaments; and a central core of homogeneous material similar to that of mature elastin. As the elastic fiber grows in size, the homogeneous material (elastin) accumulates centrally and the microfibrils are present at the periphery. With cessation of growth, the microfibril component becomes less distinct. The homogeneous component (elastin) is not believed to represent a change in physical form of the microfibrils. The microfibrils have been shown to differ in chemical composition from the homogeneous or amorphous component (elastin) on the one hand and, on the other, from collagen [238]. The exact role of microfibrils in the formation of elastin is uncertain. For the morphologist, the presence of microfibrils in elastic fibers indicates that the elastic tissue is 'young'.

Media

General features distinguishing elastic from muscular arteries were outlined in the first part of this section. The only cells found in the media of normal mammalian arteries are smooth muscle. The size and shape of arterial medial smooth muscle cells varies from species to species and with the degree of contraction of the vessel. The size of the cell increases with the increasing size of species. In the relaxed state, the cell is spindle-shaped or fusiform in section: in the contracted state, it appears to be cylindrical or rectangular in section [229]. The centrally placed nucleus is elongated in the direction of the long axis of the cell. The contour of the nucleus varies with the degree of contraction of the cell. In those cells that appear contracted, the nuclear membrane is folded and often appears 'picket fenced'. In the relaxed state, the nucleus has a smooth contour. The nucleus typically shows a zone of heterochromatin along the inner aspect of the nuclear membrane, euchromatin concentrated in the central portion, and one to two nucleoli. The tapering ends of the cell terminate in a variable number of blunt cytoplasmic processes that abut on similar processes of adjacent smooth muscle cells. There is a regular space between the outer laminae of the plasma membranes of two adjacent cells that measures approximately 100–200 Å [218, 229]. The extending cytoplasmic processes of medial smooth cells are short in the muscular arteries [218, 229]. There is no evidence of cytoplasmic continuity between smooth muscle cells in arteries, nor are specialized attachments resembling desmosomes present. Recently, however, circumscribed regions where closely related plasma membranes merged their outer leaflets to produce five layered membranes were observed between adjacent smooth muscle cells in the media of growing [39] and aging [40] rats; these 'nexus' regions are similar to those of intestinal smooth muscle cells [49]. Some consider such regions to be important in producing anatomical and functional continuity between smooth muscle cells, thus ensuring an efficient means for spread of excitation [49], essential in the absence of nerve endings in the media. The plasma membrane of smooth muscle cells in elastic arteries often closely approximates elastic plates or fibers. The area of approximation may show an apparent fusion of the basement membrane of the smooth muscle cell with the elastic fibers [197], or may appear as an electron-lucid space measuring 100–200 Å [148, 218]. Whether such areas of smooth muscle and elastic fiber approximation represent a firm attachment is unknown. The differences in appearance of the apparent junction that have been recorded may be due to differences in tissue preparation. The attachments of vascular smooth muscle appear to be to adjacent smooth muscle. Whether elastic fibers or plates also represent a definite site of attachment has not been established.

The plasma membrane of smooth muscle cells is ensheathed by a basement membrane [213], except in areas where cytoplasmic processes of adjacent smooth muscle cells are approximated. This cellular basement membrane is thinner in elastic than in muscular arteries or arterioles [213]. It is composed of moderately electron-dense flocculent-appearing material, but in man and some animal species, fine parallel filaments arranged obliquely or tangentially to the cellular surface have been observed [113, 115, 118]. The plasma membrane of smooth muscle cells displays numerous micropinocytotic vesicles, except in areas where the plasma membranes of adjacent cells are apposed. The number of micropinocytotic vesicles has been observed to be greater in smooth muscle cells of muscular than elastic arteries [218] (fig. 1, 2).

The cytoplasm of the normal smooth muscle cell is filled with thin filaments, referred to as myofilaments, aligned in the direction of the long axis of the cell. The reported thickness of these filaments varies from 4 to 30 nm. It does not appear that the thickness differs a great deal between species; according to the more recent reports, the range of thickness is 8–10 nm [229]. In only one study was an attempt made to measure the length of the myofilament; in the mouse, this was estimated to be about 1 μm [229]. The filaments are approximately 20 nm apart. Distributed in what appears to be a random arrangement in the cytoplasm are numerous electron-dense spindle-shaped areas, measuring approximately 70–400 nm in length into which the myofilaments converge. Similar electron-dense areas in the cytoplasm are adjacent to the plasma membrane; these generally are triangular in shape with the apex pointing into the cytoplasm and the base resting on the plasma membrane [219]. Myofilaments also converge into these dense areas adjacent to the plasma membrane. The electron-dense areas in the cytoplasm are composed of an amorphous material, apparently not a contractile protein, and myofilaments [229]. It has been proposed that these electron-dense areas in the cytoplasm are sites of attachment of myofilaments [219], perhaps analogous to Z-bands in striated muscle. Medial smooth muscle cells of elastic arteries are reported to have fewer electron-dense areas in the cytoplasm than those in muscular arteries [218] (fig. 1, 2).

The cytoplasm of normal vascular smooth muscle cells has very few organelles except myofilaments. Mitochondria, endoplasmic reticulum, clusters of glycogen granules, and Golgi membranes are found adjacent to the nucleus. The few profiles of endoplasmic reticulum seen in vascular smooth muscle are primarily of the granular type. Occasional electron-dense, homogeneous inclusions are seen in smooth muscle cytoplasm that appear to be lipofuscin (fig. 2).

The media of the avian elastic artery differs from that of mammalian by the presence of cells between the lamina of smooth muscle and elastic fibers that are not identifiable as smooth muscle. Muscular arteries of the avian species, however, contain only smooth muscle cells. The cells between the laminae of smooth muscle and elastic fibers in elastic arteries have been referred to as 'interlamellar connective tissue cells' [197]. These cells are stellate in shape with long processes of cytoplasm that extend for considerable distances from the cell body. The cell has no basement membrane, forms no cell-to-cell junctions with smooth muscle, and the plasma membrane shows very few micropinocytotic vesicles. Myofilaments are not seen in the cytoplasm, although there often are found arrays of filaments that resemble myofilaments. Cytoplasmic vacuoles are sometimes seen that appear to be lipid-containing. Cytoplasmic organelles including mitochondria, profiles of granular endoplasmic reticulum, Golgi apparatus, and glycogen particles have no characteristics or organization that distinguish this cell. The cell resembles a fibroblast except that cisternae of granular endoplasmic reticulum which are so characteristically found in fibroblasts are not commonly seen.

The structure of the abdominal segment of the aorta of avian species differs from that of mammalian having the appearance of a muscular artery (smooth muscle cells with a few elastic fibers). The outer portion of the media is composed of laminae of elastica, smooth muscle cells, and interlamellar connective tissue cells [197].

The distinguishing characteristics of smooth muscle cells are a limiting basement membrane, numerous micropinocytotic vesicles along the plasma membrane, and cytoplasmic myofilaments associated with the characteristic areas of cytoplasmic electron density. These characteristics considered as criteria are used by all morphologists for identification of smooth muscle. The presence of myofilaments and the characteristic zones of cytoplasmic electron density are the most conclusive criteria for cell identification, but the former can be confused with cytoplasmic tonofilaments which many cells contain. In abnormal states, these morphological characteristics are present to variable degrees resulting in uncertainties of identification. We are in need of more conclusive criteria for identification of smooth muscle cells. Histochemical technics have thus far not disclosed any reaction that characterizes smooth muscle from endothelium [128] or other cells. Immunological identification of myosin is a possible method but is technically difficult, and the absence of a reaction in a given cell will not rule out the possibility that it is a smooth muscle cell, as the filaments could be present in a portion of the cytoplasm not in the plane of section being examined. At present, we must rely for cell identification on the presence or absence of cytoplasmic myofilaments identified morphologically.

Arterial Development and Reaction to Injury

Cytological and connective tissue changes occurring during development of arteries in the embryo have been the subject of several investigations. The endothelium of fetal aorta has been observed to contain more numerous profiles of endoplasmic reticulum and mitochondria than does endothelium of adult aorta [158]. The primitive smooth muscle cell in the media is globular in shape, has few if any myofilaments, and contains numerous mitochondria and profiles of rough endoplasmic reticulum in the form of cisternae containing moderately electron-dense flocculent-appearing material [145, 146]. With maturation, the myofilaments appear and increase in number. The developing smooth muscle cell changes from a cell having the appearance of a fibroblast, including the absence of a basement membrane, to one with few cytoplasmic organelles, other than myofilaments and a limiting basement membrane [145]. Elastic tissue accumulates in the media of the developing aorta in the manner described previously – appearance of parallel arrays of microfibrils and subsequent appearance of amorphous elastin. The medial elastin of the embryo has been observed to stain differently from mature elastin by reacting positively to the periodic acid Schiff stain and metachromatic staining with toluidine blue [217]. These staining reactions correlate with the presence of microfibrils in the elastic tissue of the embryo; microfibrils are infrequent or absent in elastin of the newborn rat which does not give a positive periodic acid Schiff reaction, nor stain metachromatically with toluidine blue [217]. The elastic fibers in the media of the newborn rat aorta are thinner and smoother in contour than elastic fibers in the adult aorta [217]. There is very sparse collagen in the aorta of the newborn rat [217].

The intima and media of normal and abnormal arteries occasionally may contain vesicles up to several microns in diameter that are membrane-bound and contain varying numbers of small vesicles in an otherwise electron-lucid background (fig. 8). The nature and significance of these structures is unknown. It has been suggested that they are swollen pseudopodia of smooth muscle cells or endothelium and indicate cell injury [129].

Many methods have been used to study the cytological reaction of arteries to injury. These methods include mechanical injury [103, 130, 140, 204, 225], insertion of prostheses [48, 68, 87, 210, 267], freezing [103], lathyrism [147], embolism [266]. renal failure [254], metacorticoid hypertension [243], hyperkinetic pulmonary hypertension [63], and chemical injury [143]. If the endothelium is interrupted, a thrombus forms and the adjacent endothelium proliferates extending over the thrombus. With any type of vascular wall injury, the smooth muscle cells react with a change in their structure and undoubtedly a change in their function. The smooth muscle cells change morphologically into what has been described as 'modified smooth muscle cells'. These cells are smaller than normal smooth muscle and have an ovoid or stellate rather than fusiform shape. Cytoplasmic processes from modified smooth muscle cells are thick and extend only for short distances from the cell body in contrast to the thin and long processes of fibroblasts. The modified smooth muscle cell usually has a partial limiting basement membrane. The number of micropinocytotic vesicles in the plasma membrane usually is less than that observed in medial smooth muscle cells. The cytoplasm shows a marked increase in the numbers of mitochondria and profiles of endoplasmic reticulum relative to total cytoplasmic area and area containing myofilaments over that observed in normal smooth muscle. Myofilaments can be so reduced in number as to be evident only in a narrow zone near the plasma membrane. When the number of myofilaments is markedly reduced, the criterion for cell identification may not be too convincing. Considerable controversy has arisen with regard to cell identification in atherosclerotic lesions and will be discussed subsequently. There can be no question in the forms of arterial injury listed previously that the cells reacting to the injury are smooth muscle cells. The source of the modified smooth muscle cells, especially in prostheses, has been a subject of debate. There are three possible sources – medial smooth muscle, an undifferentiated cell from the blood, and endothelium. The endothelium as a source of modified smooth muscle cells has the least supporting evidence. It is generally true that the accumulation of modified smooth muscle cells is greater immediately beneath the endothelium than in the deeper parts of the intima. Proximity to endothelium and superficial resemblance to endothelium in terms of cytoplasmic structures is probably the best evidence that endothelium might be the origin of modified smooth muscle cells. An impressive body of evidence has accumulated with studies of prostheses in arteries, suggesting that there are cells circulating in the blood that can enter the tissue and differentiate into modified smooth muscle and perhaps normal smooth muscle cells [87, 210, 266, 267]. Recent studies with labelled cells and carefully collected blood have cast considerable doubt that there are cells in the blood that can differentiate into cells capable of elaborating connective tissue [103, 184, 225, 239, 262] and thus have a function like smooth muscle. POOLE *et al.* [225], in an excellent study and analysis of the literature, have concluded that endothelium derives from endothelium and smooth muscle derives from smooth muscle. A recent study has shown that cholesterol feeding for as short a period as three days stimulates mitotic division of normal medial smooth muscle cells [162], indicating that in experimental atherosclerosis the source of the increased smooth muscle cells is medial smooth muscle cells. A further finding of interest in this study is that normal or mature smooth muscle cells were observed in mitotic division, suggesting that smooth muscle cells need not necessarily dedifferentiate into modified smooth muscle cells prior to dividing. This finding confirms the forecasting observation by LANGHANS [159] and MCMILLAN and DUFF [182] as discussed in chapter II. In tissue culture, smooth muscle cells dedifferentiate prior to division [72].

IV. Diffuse Intimal Thickening

General Considerations

In keeping with the aims of this Monograph (see chapt. I), it appeared important to us to review the subject of diffuse intimal thickening (DIT) in some detail. The reviewing proved to be a trying experience for a variety of reasons. For one, the accounts on this intimal change are seldom found under the above title or (equally appropriate) under such names that refer to intimal (or arterial) changes in developing and growing man (or animals). Instead, information that is relevant (knowingly or unknowingly by the given authors) to this subject may be found under a multitude of other titles most of which are inaccurate and misleading. For example, many articles bear a title referring to 'changes in ageing arteries' [50, 73, 163, 249], but are in fact concerned with changes beginning in fetal life that progress through infancy and childhood. Clearly, changes taking place in most individuals in early life are not those of aging (save for conditions such as progeria); rather, they should be viewed as part of growth, maturation and remodeling. Whereas it may be difficult at a certain period in the lifespan to distinguish between features of growth and those of aging, this should hardly apply to changes taking place in infancy. Descriptions of DIT may also be found in publications entitled 'sclerosis of arteries'. Included under this topic is either the DIT alone or, in addition, the subject of atherosclerosis that, for whatever reason, is preferably referred to as sclerosis [30, 168, 202, 274, 292]. Seldom distinction is made between the two in the latter case. Moreover, since some authors regard these intimal changes to represent, indeed, the early stages of atherosclerosis, descriptions of these changes may also be found under such titles as: 'L'athérome aortique des enfants' [127] or 'The early lesions of atheroma in the coronary arteries' [164]; similar titles are employed even if the author is of the opinion that the process does not represent a stage in the development of atherosclerotic lesions [183].

As long as descriptions of changes are detailed and well illustrated, the difficulty of a misleading title may be overcome; the matter becomes, however, impossible in the absence of any morphological account. This kind of difficulty may be exemplified by a publication entitled: 'A study of coronary and aortic sclerosis: incidence and degree in 5,060 consecutive postmortem examinations' [292]. The authors state: 'In order to avoid the use of descriptive terms that may be interpreted differently by different readers, we have employed the numerical system of gradation, ranging from 0 to 4. Apparent total absence of sclerosis is graded 0; very slight degree of sclerosis, 1; moderate involvement, 2; unmistakably marked sclerosis, 3; and extreme sclerosis, 4.' This is all; illustrations representative of the entity they refer to as sclerosis or of the various gradations were not included. How is one to interpret this report? What is meant by sclerosis? Disturbing is not as much the fact that this kind of a report appeared in the literature, but that many apparently authoritative writers quote it indiscriminately (exception to this is the tactful critic expressed indirectly by PRIOR and JONES [226]).

Other difficulties arise from the fact that some authors, although not subscribing to the notion that these intimal changes are atherosclerotic in nature (or early lesions of atherosclerosis), nevertheless consider these to represent *lesions,* without commitment as to the nature of these. At times, these changes are referred to as focal lesions [183] or cushions [52]. However, it has been shown, on the basis of studies of large series of arteries of various ages, that at times the earliest manifestations of this intimal change may *begin* focally or multifocally, rather than diffusely, to extend in time over much or most of the circumference of a given vessel.

Finally, and most regretfully, the credibility, on the one hand, and the value in the form, as presented, of some reports on the other, must be seriously questioned. For example, statements that the major branches of the coronary arteries of hundreds of hearts were morphologically examined in detail, must of necessity evoke a reaction of incredibility from every thoughtful pathologist, who is aware of the time and effort required to histologically examine in detail the coronary arteries of hundreds of hearts. Attesting best to careful examination is a detailed description, and the latter is missing in many of such reports.

If one considers the enormous volume of literature devoted to atherosclerosis, one is surprised to find how little attention has been devoted to the study of the organ 'where it all happens', particularly with reference to its development, postnatal growth and re-adjustment (= remodeling) to the extrauterine environment. The data on these changes are important for our understanding of arterial reactivity with special reference to the intimal cells, for herein lies perhaps the solution to the problem of atherosclerosis. Whereas we do not claim to have reviewed all there had been written on this subject, it is perhaps 'safe' to state that the present review is based on the majority of publications we are aware were written on DIT (regardless of title employed). As will be appreciated below the number of publications on this subject is rather meager!

In man, DIT has been studied morphologically most often in the coronary arteries [30, 35, 45, 52, 65–67, 81, 90, 95, 164, 168, 183, 187, 189, 193, 202, 207, 232, 234, 247, 248, 261, 284, 285, 298, 300] and aortae [3, 21, 78, 97, 113, 126, 127, 136, 138, 139, 159, 163, 178, 200, 226, 232, 249, 270, 291]; similar changes or remodeling of a diverse nature were observed in pulmonary [237, 242, 274, 287], cerebral [263], and other arteries [13, 29, 31, 50, 97, 126, 178, 186, 211, 232, 234, 245, 301] with growth and 'aging'. Changes in the content of acid mucopolysaccharides also take place in human aorta with maturation and growth [144, 173].

It is surprising to learn that very few systematic studies on developing and maturing arterial intima of animals have been carried out and reported to date, despite the fact that a great variety of species have been employed in experimental atherosclerosis; even in the textbook on histology of domestic animals, not much reference is made to the subject [275]. Of the literature published and reviewed [19, 26, 69, 89, 135, 146, 148, 154, 157, 166, 167, 177, 194, 197, 218, 290, 299, 302], the most authoritative remains the work of Kapitoline Wolkoff [299]. She studied in detail the thoracic and abdominal aorta, the right and left coronary artery, and (in most cases) the carotid and femoral arteries from the early to the later stages of life in horses, cows, monkeys, dogs, cats, rabbits, rats, and mice. Similarly detailed studies were carried out in fewer species by other investigators [19, 154, 302, 303], but most of these were reported early in the century; very little systematic work on DIT has been undertaken in recent times. Yet, this area needs to be explored. The only study concerning the evolutionary stages of the arteries (particularly intima) in pigs that has been carried out recently in great depth is that of Laing *et al.* [157]. Regretfully, the work has not been published *in toto* to date.

As employed in this Monograph and used by most contemporary pathologists, the term 'diffuse intimal thickening' refers to the thickening of arterial intima that begins early in neonatal life (and may be at times observed in fetuses) in all human beings, and progresses gradually and through well-defined stages characterized by morphologically recognizable layers over puberty to adult life. It is 'diffuse' because it involves ultimately most or the entire circumference and (in large arteries) length, although its growth may have been at first focal or multifocal. The rate with which the DIT progresses varies not only in individuals of the same age, but from one artery to another, at different levels of the same artery, and at different circumferential sites of a given artery. Whereas this process, characterized by the development of layers, is basically the same in every artery, its rate of growth and ultimate morphology is modified by the structure (and function of a given artery (and its segments); thus, it has to be studied in detail in individual arteries and at various levels thereof.

In the following account, the histogenesis of DIT in the aorta and coronary arteries of man will be considered first; these arteries were selected because a somewhat more detailed information concerning their DIT is available, and because of the important position they occupy in human atherosclerosis. Next, pertinent data on our knowledge of DIT in animals will be discussed, as these will facilitate our understanding of the possible role of DIT in terms of physiology and – if any – pathology of the arteries. Having provided the above 'background', it appears logical to consider next in detail the core of this Monograph's concern, i.e., the nature and role of the cellular elements in the DIT. An attempt at interpretation of the significance of the DIT will close the section.

Diffuse Intimal Thickening in Man

Aorta

It has been appreciated for at least one hundred years that the thickness of the aortic intima increases with age. LANGHANS [159] was impressed with the variations of intimal thickness; he carried out actual measurements on intimas of aortas obtained *post mortem* in 1866. These measurements, made on preparations of dried ascending aortas, which were subsequently immersed in diluted acetic acid, ranged from 0.015–0.02 mm in a four-day-old infant to 0.08–0.12 mm at the age of fifty years. Thereafter, the measurements varied from 0.05 to 0.12 mm. LANGHANS concentrated his efforts on studying the cellular components of the thickened intima (to be discussed in some detail later in this section). He commented on the appearance of well-definable layers in the intima at the age of ten years. He quoted the work of KÖLLIKER who, several years prior to him, drew attention to the presence of elastic tissue-rich 'layering' in the intima. In 1896, GRÜNSTEIN [97] and, in 1914, MASLOFF [178], gave detailed accounts on their morphological studies of growing human aorta, with special reference to the intima, the former in postnatal, the latter in intrauterine life, providing at the same time through reviews on the subject. However, it was largely left to JORES, in the early part of this century, to describe carefully and in detail the gradual development of the intima in a rather organized, well-systematized fashion into the ultimate stage of three layers [138, 139]. His observations were confirmed subsequently; in recent years, the morphogenesis of these layers was re-examined and found to be in accord with JORES' original descriptions [200].

In the fetus, the endothelium adheres to the internal elastic lamina and the subendothelial (intimal) space is virtually nonexistent. The same obtains usually in the newborn fullterm infant. However, it has been documented that occasionally a definite intima (usually thin and having a focal rather than diffuse character) is present at birth even in premature infants who survive for some days. JORES [138] recorded such observations, and MASLOFF quotes ASCHOFF who stated that a definite subendothelial layer may exist in human aorta in the sixth month of intrauterine life [178, p. 361]. The first change that heralds the development of the intima consists of what has been termed 'splitting' of the internal elastic lamina (IEL) on its luminal aspect. That split may be either into equally thick portions of the lamina – the inner half is then referred to as the inner limiting membrane –, or numerous thin elastic lamellae may be split off toward the subendothelial region. In either case, the process is at first largely focal and involves the entire circumference of the IEL only with progression of time. Smooth muscle cells that are believed to migrate through the naturally occurring fenestrae of the IEL, from the media into the newly broadening space between the IEL and the endothelium, appear shortly thereafter assuming a position parallel to the long axis of the vessel. These cells are intermingled with elastic lamellae that continue to split off (or so it has been said) of the IEL. Thus, the first intimal layer, the so-called musculo-elastic layer, has been established; it is usually well apparent between the age of six months to one year. In addition to its two principal components, it contains acid mucopolysaccharide-rich ground substance, but only very few and thin collagen fibers.

At the time when the musculo-elastic layer is being formed, some coarse elastic fibers split off the internal limiting membrane into the region between the latter and the endothelium, assuming a longitudinal position. This process continues and it becomes apparent that the newly split coarse fibers, in turn, give rise to other elastic fibers. Between the quickly 'multiplying' elastic fibers of this newly forming elastic-hyperplastic layer, cells appear in the outer zone, i.e., adjacent to the musculo-elastic layer, that have features and arrangement similar to those of the cells in that layer. In the inner zone of the elastic-hyperplastic layer, the cellular features are in some aspects reminiscent of fibroblasts by light microscopy (the details of the cellular components are discussed later in this chapter), and the direction and arrangement haphazard. Whereas this layer is usually present in the second decade of life, its continuous growth in width accounts largely for the increasing intimal thickness beyond this age.

In the middle decades of life and usually when the elastic-hyperplastic layer has attained a considerable thickness, a third, the innermost connective tissue layer, develops. This is the most irregularly developing layer in that it may be of a somewhat circumferential, segmental, or even more focal distribution. Usually, it does not reach the thickness of the elastic-hyperplastic layer. It consists of loosely arranged connective tissues, particularly collagen fibers and thin elastic fibers, all having a circular arrangement in contradistinction to the longitudinal direction of the fibers in the elastic-hyperplastic layer. The sparse ground substance of this layer shows little metachromasia and thus is not rich in acid mucopolysaccharides. This layer is usually present in old age; however, at times, the intima may consist of the two other layers only, even in advanced age.

The rate of growth of the individual layers varies considerably along the aorta. As a rule, the intima develops faster in the distal than in the proximal parts of the aorta, and is thinner in the latter than in the former at periods of life prior to advanced age. Differences between proximal and distal parts of the aorta are most marked and consistent from the first to the fourth decades. For example, in the third decade, the intima is quite thin in the upper thoracic aorta; in the upper abdominal segment, it may attain two to three times and, in the lower abdominal aorta, eight to ten times the thickness of the intima of the thoracic aorta [200] (fig. 4a, b). Later, the thickness of the intima may progress in the proximal aorta sufficiently to become equal to that of the distal segment. Consistent differences between the intima of ventral and dorsal portions of the vessels were not observed by some [200], but described by others [226, 291], who maintained that the dorsal aortic intima is thicker than the ventral at the same level.

Some difficulties in identification of individual layers may be encountered when the transition from one to the other is gradual rather than sharp and distinct. The best criterion for identifying the 'territory' of one versus the other layer is the direction of the elastic fibers, particularly those in the elastic-hyperplastic layer, as here they are almost always arranged in the longitudinal direction. Other difficulties of identification may obtain when

– at a variable age! – (secondary) degenerative changes begin to affect some or all elements of the DIT. Smooth muscle cells atrophy with time and either become so atrophic that most of their characteristics are no longer discernible, or they disappear. Thus, this distinguishing characteristic between the musculo-elastic and elastic-hyperplastic layers may be lost. Hyalinization of formed connective tissue fibers occurs also at different ages; it may affect fibers in various layers at approximately the same time, thus obscuring the pattern of layers. Hyalinization is most conspicuous in the connective tissue layer, but the latter is not always present (see above) or developed by the time the degenerative process sets in affecting other layers.

Areas of DIT only (i.e., intima that appears normal on gross examination), as a rule, do not show the presence of intracellular fat on microscopic examination. Extracellular fat in a finely dispersed form may be present in small amounts in early life along the elastic lamellae; it slowly increases over the third and fourth decade and is found ubiquitously, still largely along the elastic elements (fig. 4a, b).

Coronary Arteries

It is quite surprising to learn that the first description of the microscopic appearance of a human coronary artery was published in 1912 [65]. EDHOLM [65] examined 'two peripheral segments and one from the area of origin of an arteria coronaria cordis of an executed man'. He quotes KÖLLIKER'S [153] 'Handbuch der Gewebelehre des Menschen' (1902) in which mention is made of V. CALLUCCI'S report (in Mem. d. R. Accad. di Bologna, 1898) regarding the microscopic appearance of coronary arteries in domestic animals. EDHOLM was impressed by the appearance of the coronary artery, because it differed considerably from that of other arteries and in no way did the structure resemble that of the aorta. He noticed that the intima was thick and contained scattered elastic fibers that were split off the IEL. He described further what he believed were two distinct layers of the media: the inner, consisting of longitudinally arranged smooth muscle cells and numerous elastic fibers, and the outer, with these elements arranged circularly. He stressed the fact that most of the elastic tissue of the artery was concentrated in the inner layer of the media. Between the two medial layers, he observed a distinct elastic membrane with fenestrations.

It is quite apparent from the above description that EDHOLM mistook the prominent elastic-hyperplastic (and the musculo-elastic) layer of the intima for an 'inner' layer of the media, being probably reluctant to admit that an intima in an artery of the size of the coronary artery could be *that* thick. No detail regarding the age of the man, nor even which of the main coronary arteries was subjected to examination, is provided by EDHOLM.

Since this original description of the coronary arteries, other accounts with reference to the DIT appeared in the literature. The most authoritative remains that published by WOLKOFF in 1923 [298], and by GROSS *et al.* in 1934 [95]. The latter actually complemented in some respect the observations of the former, and all were again emphasized in recent years [193]

To avoid repetition, the work of WOLKOFF will be quoted and other reports cited only as they differ from the observations in the aorta, or when they pertain to observations beyond those reported for the aorta. Similarly, observations of GROSS *et al.* [95] will be quoted that were made in addition to, or were at variance with those of WOLKOFF [298].

Of all human arteries examined, the intima is thickest in the coronary arteries. Its basic structure and growth evolves in a fashion as described for the aortic intima, but this pertains largely to the main branches. The differences of rate of growth and, therefore, in part of structure are encountered at different levels of the arteries and to some extent also between the main branches at the same level. WOLKOFF examined the coronary arteries of nine[6] hearts obtained at necropsy of patients whose age ranged from eight months to fifty years. Twelve blocks removed from each heart contained the following segments of each of the three major coronary arteries: a small intramyocardial, a small subepicardial, a medium-size segment, and the main stems of each of these arteries from their origin to the point of origin of the first branch given off by the respective main artery. WOLKOFF found that the differences of arterial structure between the three main arteries, their segments and branches were largely (although *not* exclusively) confined to the intima; the same applied to changes with age. These changes were at first (i.e., in early life) almost always focal, not involving the entire circumference.

As in the aorta, the initial changes consist of splitting of the IEL and development of a musculo-elastic layer; this layer appears in infancy and is well established at the age of seven years in the main, major and medium-size branches. At the age of fifteen years, the thickness of the intima exceeds that of other arterial coats and consists invariably of two definite layers

[6] The number of hearts is being mentioned here purposely, as is the number of blocks removed from each, to document that detailed and careful studies on the morphogenesis of the intimal changes could not have been made on hundreds of hearts (as claimed in some publications!).

(musculo-elastic and elastic-hyperplastic) in the main arteries and their larger branches; at times, the connective tissue layer is present in focal areas (fig. 3). All three layers are present at the age of 18 years and are well developed in the first part of the third decade in the main arteries. At the beginning of the fourth decade, the intima with its three layers is also well developed in the medium-size branches and attains here the width of the media; in the second part of the same decade, it reaches its full growth and does not progress further. At this stage, the intima in the medium-size and even small branches shows the thickness and structure that are similar to those seen in the intima of the main arteries of the adolescent and young adult.

The intramyocardial branches of all cases examined by WOLKOFF and the subepicardial branches until the fifteenth year of life showed still the 'simple' intima, i.e., the endothelium resting upon the IEL with no space or tissue intervening. Later in life, this arrangement persisted in some areas of the circumference of the subepicardial branches, whereas in others, splitting of the IEL with focal formation of a definite intima was observed.

Finally, WOLKOFF reported that the IEL may become discontinuous in some areas of the circumference. She observed such areas in the main branches of the coronary arteries in the heart of a fifteen-year-old and stated that the entire circumference was 'affected' after the age of thirty years. Somewhat astonishing (and unexpected of her) is the statement that discontinuities and ultimate disappearance of the IEL are the consequence of 'being used up in the further formation of new elastic elements', thus timing this process until after the elastic-hyperplastic layer had been fully developed. Did she intend to indicate that the 'growth' of that layer, believed to take place at the expense of the inner limiting membrane or the equivalent thick lamellae, initially split off from the IEL, now proceeds from the outer instead of from the original inner direction? If so, how do these elastic elements 'reach' the elastic-hyperplastic layer, by 'crossing' the musculo-elastic layer? The matter of the disappearance of the IEL will be discussed below, based on the work of GROSS *et al.* [95].

If one follows intimal development with age in the direction from the smallest (intramyocardial) to the largest branches with WOLKOFF, one may summarize by stating that the DIT progresses with the size of the artery; when achieving its full growth-potential in the largest branches, it is seen in the intramyocardial branches still as a simple intima (endothelium on IEL); in the subepicardial branches as foci of musculo-elastic layer, developing between the IEL and the inner limiting membrane split focally off the latter; and in the medium-size branches consisting of a well-developed musculo-elastic layer and an elastic-hyperplastic layer in various stages of development (as a result of splitting of elastic fibers from the inner limiting membrane with disappearance of the latter in many areas). In larger branches, the thickness of the elastic-hyperplastic layer increases considerably, the inner limiting membrane disappears entirely, and, in addition, the innermost connective tissue layer develops focally. In the main arteries, the intima is thickest owing to increases in width of both the elastic-hyperplastic and connective tissue layers until the beginning of the fourth decade; in addition, the IEL that showed areas of discontinuity in these arterial segments at an earlier age, disappears entirely, no longer allowing for a sharp delineation of the intima from media.

The structural differences between the intima of the right and that of the left coronary arteries are appreciated best in the main stems of the arteries: The connective tissue layer is thinner in the left than right coronary artery, but the reverse is true with respect to the two other layers, as these are always thicker in the left than in the right coronary artery.

Observations on additional structural components of the developing DIT in the coronary arteries made by GROSS *et al.* [95] are important not only for the academic reason of achieving completeness, but because these may explain certain physiological and perhaps also pathological characteristics of these arteries. These observations concern largely the border area between the intima and media and may be summarized, also on the basis of another study [193], as follows:

At some time during the process of splitting of the IEL, discontinuities in the latter creating true gaps may occur. At times, this phenomenon may be observed as early as in the third month of life and is found usually in either of the two main branches of the left artery. This gap formation was termed 'border disappearance' by GROSS *et al.* [95]. At the same time, or at a later stage, both the intima and media contribute longitudinally arranged bundles of smooth muscle cells that occupy the areas of the border disappearance and give rise to a new, so-called intermediary layer; in addition to smooth muscle cells, this new layer contains fine elastic fibrils closely applied to cells. The smooth muscle cells 'contributed' by the intima are derived from the musculo-elastic layer; these maintain their longitudinal direction, whereas those derived from the media have to change their position from circular to longitudinal. With time, the number of border disappearances increases and becomes 'confluent', that is, the IEL disappears gradually, its position being occupied by fusion of individual areas of the intermediary layer now expanding circumferentially. Moreover, the intermediary layer grows in width and, at times, attains a considerable thickness. But as in the case of the other intimal layers, it varies widely from one individual to another and from one artery or arterial segment to another. Whereas in some individuals it develops quite early, i.e., at a time when there is only a musculo-elastic layer present, it may be entirely absent in others, even in the coronary arteries of adults and despite the presence of the 'border disappearance'. At times, this layer occupies almost the entire circumference of a vessel as early as at the end of the first decade.

A curious phenomenon may be at times observed in the media subjacent to the IEL: Bundles composed of a few muscle cells having a distinct longitudinal arrangement are observed in the immediate vicinity of an intact IEL. Whether with time these bundles will become a component of an intermediary layer is not known and probably depends primarily on the formation of a gap in this immediately adjacent area of the IEL. The intermediary layer is present in the left descending and circumflex arteries more often than in the right.

There is practically no information on the function and potentials of this intermediary layer. Is it designed to substitute more efficiently for the role of the IEL, which cannot be fulfilled in arteries of a medium size, but which is exposed to extremely high blood pressures and flow patterns imposed by the episodic contractions and dilations of the organ they supply? Are the stimuli for the contraction of the smooth muscle cells of this layer the same as those for the medial cells? If they are, it appears that this layer would allow for an elongation of the particular segment without reducing the diameter of the artery.

The field for investigation of the architecture, detailed structure, and function of this layer under normal and pathological conditions is wide open.

Diffuse Intimal Thickening in Animals

It has been maintained in some publications – putting forth arguments in support of the view that the DIT is either a forerunner or an early lesion of atherosclerosis – that this intimal change is confined to man and does not exist in the animal kingdom [291]. This is not correct; for, while it is true that very few systematic studies have been reported on the structural changes taking place in the arteries of animals from early to late stages of life, the publications that are available on the subject document that DIT occurs also in animals.

It is beyond the scope of this Monograph to discuss in detail the DIT as reported in the literature for various species and different arteries. Interested readers are referred to excellent accounts – few as they may be – provided at the beginning of this century, along with a thorough review of the available literature by BAUM and THIENEL [19], who reported in 1904 on their examination of the arteria axillaris in horse, donkey, cow, calf, sheep, pig, and dog; by ZINSERLING [302], who reported in 1913 on the morphology of equine aorta; by KRAUSE [154], who published the most extensive review on the subject in 1922, when he reported his morphological observations on intimal changes with age in aortas of horses, cows and dogs; and by WOLKOFF [299]. WOLKOFF chose the thoracic and abdominal aorta, the right and left coronary arteries (main trunks, medium-size and subepicardial branches) and, in most cases, the carotid and femoral arteries from early to late stages of life of horses, cows, monkeys, dogs, cats, rabbits, rats, and mice. The unique value of her work is not only the thoughtful detail and meticulous care with which she examined these changes, but, in addition, her wise choice of species from smallest to largest.

Information regarding certain other species may be found in the above-quoted references; more recent data are available on pigs [69, 70, 135, 157], dogs [166, 194][7], monkeys [89, 167][7] and other species [26, 148, 218], as also indicated in the general considerations of this chapter.

Our concern here is to summarize the changes that take place in animals with age, and compare these with changes occurring in man, in an attempt at correlating the extent of the DIT with factors that may possibly be relevant.

It may be stated that the arterial intima increases in thickness with age in all animals examined, although in the smallest (mice, rats) these changes were either not present (by light microscopy) or became apparent only in very advanced age [299]. By electron microscopy, older mice and rats showed consistently thicker intima or 'wider subendothelial space', containing a variety of components, than did the younger animals [146, 148, 218]. The intimal thickening begins at different times and progresses at different rates from species to species and from one artery to another. In a given artery, it begins in the proximal segment and, with time, progresses distally; but there is evidence that this rule may not apply to the aorta of the pig. Some data indicate that with age the thickness of the intima in the pig abdominal seg-

[7] These authors do not refer actually to the changes described as DIT, and some consider these to be part of atherosclerosis. However, the intimal alterations described are consistent with those of diffuse thickening rather than atherosclerosis.

ment exceeds that in the thoracic segment; whereas in one study, the aortic intima was as thick in the proximal part of the thoracic segment as it was in the distal abdominal segment of the vessel [157]. This problem has not been clarified definitely.

Morphologically, DIT results from the formation of the musculo-elastic layer that begins with splitting of the IEL and increases with age, the development of an inner connective tissue layer at more advanced age, and a gradual accumulation of ground substance. The development of the musculo-elastic layer in the aorta takes place much earlier and considerably faster than in the coronary arteries, and was observed in larger animals even in intrauterine life. WOLKOFF [299] reported that this phenomenon occurred in the ascending aorta of a two-month-old equine fetus and a seven-month-old cow fetus; KRAUSE [154] observed that the IEL was replaced in the aorta by a musculo-elastic layer in horses, cows and dogs in the second half of fetal life. WOLKOFF observed the presence of this layer in the aorta of a newborn puppy, an eight-day-old cat, and a two-week-old rabbit.

In coronary arteries, development of DIT 'trails' behind that of aortic DIT in time, extent and width, and appears for example in such animals as cats, dogs and monkeys only in young adult life; in the rabbit, it was observed as late as at the age of three years, and only in the left coronary artery [299]. In smaller and medium-sized animals (rabbit, cat, dog and monkey), the DIT is largely, although not exclusively, localized in the vicinity of the origins of the main arteries, whereas in large animals (cow and horse), the DIT extends to the level of medium-size branches; however, it does not reach the small subepicardial branches.

There appears to be no consistency with respect to the occurrence of a connective tissue layer, as no definite correlation could be ascertained between the observations regarding this layer and data pertaining to age of animals, location, extent of involvement and type of arteries. WOLKOFF stated that perhaps there is an association of this layer with age, but that other factors characteristic of the animals themselves influence the development of this layer most. No definite sex difference within a given animal species has been reported.

On the basis of all information available to date, it is correct to state that the extent of the DIT is directly associated only with the size of the given animal. In other words, the intima grows in width as the animal grows in length (and therefore the arteries, too). Apparently, there is no relation between the intensity of work performed by the animals and the extent of the DIT [299].

In spite of the similarities that exist between the DIT in man and animals, there are also fundamental differences; these pertain largely to the overall architecture of the DIT and to the rate of growth in various arteries and in different segments. The DIT of animals is architecturally simpler than that in man, as it consists of the musculo-elastic layer and later acquires the inner connective tissue layer to a quite variable extent. A notable exception to this rule has been reported for the pig: the two zones distinguished in the DIT were likened to the elastic-hyperplastic and musculo-elastic layer in man [69]. This observation awaits confirmation. It may be that the layer designated by the above workers as elastic-hyperplastic was considered by others to represent the connective tissue layer. Thus, the prominent elastic-hyperplastic layer of human DIT does not exist. Since the musculo-elastic layer in animals is richer in coarse (and numerous) elastic fibers than is the same layer in man, KRAUSE [154] was inclined to believe that, in animals, it represents a composite of both the musculo-elastic and elastic-hyperplastic layers of DIT of man; it is the result of a fast growth of the given animal; growth occurs in a much shorter time and for a shorter lifespan than the growth of man. The other fundamental difference concerns the rate of growth and the extent of the DIT in aorta versus the coronary arteries. In man, the width of the intima in the coronary arteries exceeds ultimately the thickness of the media; but this does not happen in animals, even in those in whom the development of the DIT begins earlier than in man. And finally, with the possible exception of the pig, the DIT of growing and maturing aorta in animals is better developed in the proximal than distal segments, whereas the reverse prevails in man at the time he reaches the middle and later part of life. Many other rather subtle differences exist between the various animal species on the one hand and man on the other, but these do not appear to be of a fundamental nature and importance.

Cellular Elements in Diffuse Intimal Thickening

Study of the nature and properties of cells in the DIT is important, because it is reasonable to assume that factors applying to conditions of normal growth and maturation of the intima will shed light on the behavior of the intimal cells in atherosclerosis. It is postulated by this approach that the cells involved in atherosclerosis derive from the cellular population of the DIT, but this does not exclude the probability that, in addition, other cells may participate in this pathological process of the intima.

Again, as is true with most subjects considered in this Monograph, the matter of cellular elements in DIT has not been clarified entirely to date, as only the cells of one, the musculo-elastic layer, have been identified and characterized unequivocally. That they are smooth muscle cells was obvious, even to those earliest investigators who first described and named this layer. Nevertheless, it became apparent to them, too, that these cells differ morphologically somewhat from similar cells of the media on the one hand, and on the other from those observed in the atherosclerotic lesions (see chapt. II).

Identity of cells in other layers has not been the subject of intense investigation, and with one exception [78] it is usually dealt with in a rather superficial manner. The importance of cells in intima was recognized by LANGHANS [159], who directed his examination of the DIT largely towards the identity of cells. Provided one interprets his long deliberations on morphology correctly, an interesting concept emerges that may explain the diverse appearance of possibly only one cell type in the intima. Thus, in all intimas of the ascending human aorta examined by LANGHANS, the shape and number of extensions of the spindle or star-like intimal cells was directly related to the 'mass' of extracellular connective tissue components present in the mesh between the interconnecting (?) extensions of these cells. It is logical that with the expansion of the extracellular components, the cellular extensions become narrower and fewer, the cellular body more slender, and the staining quality of the nucleoproteins altered – all features that may lead to the interpretation that a variety of cells are present in the DIT, rather than recognizing that these may represent different (functional) stages of the same basic cell. Thus it is understandable that, in the areas outside the musculo-elastic layer, the cells have been regarded variously as smooth muscle cells with a few fibroblasts and histiocytes [200], only fibroblasts [225], or mast cells, macrophages, monocytes, lymphocytes, fibroblasts and smooth muscle cells all at once [200]. Other authors accommodated their opinion anywhere between these three extremes.

Intimal thickening has not been studied intensively by electron microscopists in man, and we must draw upon rather limited observations in human aorta for further characterization of the cells [78]. Near the IEL, the cells in the thickened intima are typical large smooth muscle, identified by the usual criteria of limiting basement membrane, numerous micropinocytotic vesicles along the plasma membrane, and abundant myofilaments in the cytoplasm. Near the endothelium, a variety of cells may be distinguished morphologically. For purposes of description, we will consider three general types that appear to be rather distinct. Whether these cells have a common progenitor or represent truly different cells is unknown at present.

One cell is largely ovoid in shape and morphologically indistinguishable from a blood monocyte. It usually is located very close to the endothelium, but no definite relation between these two cells was observed. The cell has no basement membrane. The plasma membrane shows very few micropinocytotic vesicles. Short microvillous extensions of the cytoplasm into the surrounding connective tissue space are frequently present. The cytoplasm contains few organelles; these include primarily agranular endoplasmic reticulum, mitochondria, and free ribonucleoprotein granules. The nucleus usually is kidney-shaped and contains a single nucleolus and large areas of heterochromatin (this cell type is depicted in fig. 15–17).

The second cell type found in thickened intima varies considerably in shape and organelle content. Since in general this cell conforms to what is widely regarded as modified smooth muscle, we are considering that the rather wide range of appearances represents a single cell type of varying degrees of differentiation. This consideration is not necessarily valid. The cell shape varies from elongate to stellate to ovoid; this variation may at least in part be due to different planes of section, e.g., a fusiform cell sectioned in its midportion and viewed on end would appear as a round cell. The cytoplasmic to nuclear ratio varies widely. Cytoplasmic processes extending into the surrounding connective tissue space, when present, are broad or thick and reach out for only short distances from the cell body. The plasma membrane contains a variable number of micropinocytotic vesicles. At least a portion of the plasma membrane of most of these cells possesses an adjacent basement membrane. Some such cells have a complete basement membrane. The nucleus is variable in shape and typically shows a thin condensed border of chromatin adjacent to the nuclear membrane. The cytoplasm contains scattered mitochondria, profiles of granular endoplasmic reticulum, and free ribonucleoprotein granules. Cisternae of granular endoplasmic reticulum are frequently present and contain a moderately electron-dense flocculent-appearing material. The cytoplasm may contain scattered small filaments resembling myofilaments of smooth muscle cells; sometimes areas of electron density are seen that are identical to those among myofilaments in smooth muscle cells. The filaments resembling myofilaments usually are adjacent to the plasma membrane. This cell differs from the typical smooth muscle cell by being smaller in size, having more numerous cytoplasmic organelles relative to cytoplasmic area, and far fewer cytoplasmic filaments. The cell resembles smooth muscle more than does the first cell type, or the one to be described in the next paragraph. The resemblance of this cell to smooth muscle cells in the arteries of experimental animals reacting to a variety of injuries is unmistakable; it may be thus assumed that the modified smooth muscle cell is derived from smooth muscle (fig. 9–11).

The third cell type found in human thickened aortic intima differs morphologically considerably from the two cell types described above. It has been observed only in infants [78]. This cell is indistinguishable by any criteria we know from a fibroblast. The cell is stellate in configuration with thin, long cytoplasmic processes extending into the surrounding connective tissue space. There is no limiting basement membrane. Very few micropinocytotic vesicles are present along the plasma membrane. There is scant cytoplasm in the cell body, which shows cisternae of granular endoplasmic reticulum containing a moderately electron-dense flocculent-appearing material (fig. 8). Recalling the maturation of fibroblast-like cells in the aorta of chick embryos to typical smooth muscle cells, it may be postulated that the former differentiate in the intima of infants through various stages into typical smooth muscle cells. There are too few observations recorded to allow for more than speculation on this point.

Significance of Diffuse Intimal Thickening

The main points of contention regarding DIT may be summarized as follows: (a) Is the DIT an integral part of atherosclerotic lesions; (b) if a does not apply, how should this intimal change be viewed (i.e., as another form of arterial lesion or a normal developmental process); and (c) if a does not apply, does the DIT predispose to the formation of atherosclerotic lesions? It is not possible to consider each of the above issues separately, as the evidence and arguments in support of one overlap the territory of the others, and will thus have to be discussed jointly.

Jores, who contributed much to our knowledge on the subject, considered the DIT to be a normal development, as it affected all individuals. In support of his interpretations, he also pointed out the fact that the rate with which this thickening develops, for example in the human aorta, is fastest in the first three decades of life, i.e., during the actual period of rapid arterial growth, and therefore paralleling this growth. To this period he refers as the 'first or ascending period of vascular growth' ('erste oder aufsteigende Periode des Gefässwachstums'). This development is followed by a second period extending into the middle or end of the fourth decade, during which no considerable further growth or change occurs in the DIT; this period may therefore be regarded as a stationary period. During a third or declining period ('absteigende Periode'), collagenization and some increase in intimal thickening are thought to take place [139]. Similar schemes of growth periods apply to the intima of human coronary arteries; but the times are different because the rates of growth differ from those in the aorta (see above). There are other data to support the view that the DIT represents a normal growth of the intima as an integral part of arterial growth and remodeling. Contrary to some statements made in the literature [291], DIT has been observed in all mammalian species examined with care, even in those of smallest size in which no such alteration was appreciated by light microscopy [299]; evidence for developing DIT with age in these species, was provided by electron microscopic studies [146, 148, 218], and the following statement was made: 'We have seen this (i.e., the developing of various connective tissue components in the wide subendothelial space and protrusions of smooth muscle cells from the media through fenestrations of the IEL) as such a common feature of aortic structure (of rats) that we do not regard it as in any way pathological' [218].

Of great importance appears to be the fact that the degree of DIT with age is related to the actual size of a given animal species and *not* to the tendency to develop atherosclerosis; animals such as the dog and baboon, which develop more diffuse thickening than the pig, show less propensity for development of atherosclerosis than the latter. It is also noteworthy that the greater the width of the DIT in a given species, the earlier the development of the DIT begins; in the horse and cow, this development begins early in fetal life. Thus, if the DIT is a feature of all mammal species examined to date and is present in all members within a given species, it begins in intrauterine life in larger-size species and achieves the greatest thickness in largest animal species (is therefore size-related); but as the thickness does not correlate with the propensity of a given species to develop atherosclerosis, it is difficult to accept the view that the DIT is an integral part of atherosclerosis. Some, who suggest this, go as far as to propose: '... atherosclerosis is not a process that is limited to scattered areas of the arterial intima but is one that involves the entire intima'; further, 'Diffuse intimal thickening (of the aorta) does not occur in species that do not develop atherosclerosis spontaneously' [291]. The latter statement is not correct, as may be seen from the review in this chapter.

Those who believe the DIT to be a part of the atherosclerotic process quote work in support of differences in sex and race that correlate with the degree of the DIT. From these data, it would appear that in male subjects the thickness exceeds that of female subjects, whether it be in the coronary arteries [52, 67] or aorta [226, 291]. Since the incidence of atherosclerosis is greater in men than women, the proponents of the theory see a direct correlation between these data. However, other studies do not indicate (directly or indirectly) such correlation in man [168, 200, 247], and certainly there is no evidence from studies in animals to support it. Similarly, one may quote the pros and cons with respect to ethnic groups or race, but few investigations have been undertaken to study this problem. In one report, data are provided to show that differences exist between three ethnic groups in the same country with respect to the extent of the DIT; this apparently correlates well with the incidence of atherosclerosis in each group [285]. On the basis of some photomicrographs provided and various statements made, it is difficult to accept the data and conclusions as presented in this publication. Further detailed work is needed in this area. Moreover, in another study designed to test whether intimal thickenings occur in the arteries of African infants and how they compare with those of European and North American subjects, it was shown that the incidence and degree of intimal thickening and elastic reduplication (in the coronary and popliteal arteries) is similar in all groups [234]. Since atherosclerosis is much less severe and extensive in the African Bantu and Negro than in Europeans, the author concluded that the presence of the intimal thickening plays little part in determining the later development of atherosclerosis [234].

It would therefore, appear that most facts support the view that the DIT is not an integral part of atherosclerotic lesions, or – phrased differently – insufficient data are available at present to show that the DIT represents a stage in atherosclerosis.

How should then the DIT be viewed? From many arguments put forward above, it does appear equally unlikely that it represents yet another form of arterial lesions; the bulk of evidence favors the view that it is the outcome (or component) of arterial growth and remodeling. This intimal growth does not seem to be incidental to the vascular growth, but rather is the result of a functional need dictated perhaps by the necessity to either replace or complement the action of the IEL in a growing organism. There are many factors that have bearing upon the vascular growth and remodeling (and thus directly or indirectly upon the DIT). It is beyond the ambition of this Monograph to discuss these, and interested readers are instead referred to an uniquely competent, exciting and thorough review on this subject written by Baden [13].

There remains the question whether or not the DIT, itself a normal phenomenon, predisposes to the development of atherosclerosis. Those who favor this idea cite studies showing that arteries with minimal DIT are usually not the site of atherosclerotic lesions [245], whereas those with prominent DIT are most commonly involved [291]. Similarly, they interpret the observation that hypertension apparently is associated with a greater extent and degree of DIT on the one hand [291] and with accelerated atherosclerosis on the other [91, 216 233] by assuming the former influences the latter. Moreover, the sites of predilection for the development of atherosclerosis are reportedly those where the greatest width of the DIT is found. Conversely, one could argue that the DIT is entirely unrelated to the inception and progression of at least certain forms of atherosclerotic lesions, as fatty dots and streaks may be observed in the aorta at an age at which the diffuse thickening is either not apparent at all or very minimal. One could also interpret the observations quoted above differently and postulate that there are certain factors, e.g., hypertension and other hemodynamic factors, that influence the rate and extent of development of the DIT as well as atherosclerotic lesions. This interpretation is quite reasonable in view of the fact that certainly hemodynamic factors (among others) are thought to influence the growth and remodeling of arteries [13] and, through these, the development of the DIT. Some experimental data implicate feeding of a high fat diet in the development of DIT [46, 134, 162]; the mechanism for induction of cellular proliferation and intimal thickening with a high fat diet is unknown, but again this would be another factor common to both, the DIT and (experimentally produced) atherosclerosis. From a purely speculative point of view, it is quite conceivable that many factors that may produce DIT, when acting 'on purposeful demand', will be or may become instrumental in the genesis or progression of atherosclerotic lesions, outside the physiological limits (either in time, intensity, or localization); this would certainly apply to some hemodynamic factors (hypertension).

Finally, it has to be admitted that nourishing and clearing the intima of waste products or substances that entered from the blood not by physiological 'intention', becomes more difficult with increasing thickness of the avascular intima. When, in addition, collagenization and hyalinization of the thickened intima occurs in later life, these problems become exaggerated and thus, logically, accumulation of fat derived from blood, degeneration of local connective tissue and cellular elements, edema and other changes may herald the development of atherosclerotic lesions. There is experimental evidence that a thickened intima is more susceptible to lipid desposition than is normal intima [38, 129, 195, 198, 290].

There must be, however, other factors acting simultaneously to localize the lesion to certain areas [91]; were the thickened or hyalinized intima alone responsible for the development of atherosclerosis, it would be diffusely rather than focally involved. That the problem of adequate nourishment is a factor in atherosclerosis and no doubt also in the degenerative phenomena in the thickened intima, is exemplified by the abdominal aorta in man where both the DIT is most pronounced and atherosclerosis severest. As has been emphasized recently [295], no vasa vasorum penetrate the media of abdominal aorta in man; thus, the conditions for diffusion and mural nourishment must of necessity be less favorable here than in the thoracic segment in which the vasa vasorum penetrate the outer third of the media.

It is quite apparent that innumerable aspects of the DIT need to be explored further in investigations that should be carefully planned and competently executed.

V. Early Lesions of Atherosclerosis

As indicated in chapter II, in recent years two facts have been established that are relevant to the role of smooth muscle cells in atherosclerotic lesions: these cells accumulate fat and are a prominent feature in grossly visible fatty dots and streaks; in addition, they are the cellular element in the fibrous plaque (devoid of, or containing, an atheroma) responsible for connective tissue production. It therefore appears that it would suffice to limit our discussion to the two forms of atherosclerotic lesions, i.e., the fatty dots and streaks, and fibrous plaques. This approach, however, would serve no meaningful purpose because it would take into consideration only segments of a complex pathobiological process, instead of viewing smooth muscle cells in the context of the entire gamut of tissue reactions that operate in this disease. Admittedly, we do not know whether smooth muscle cells play a role also in the evolution of other forms of atherosclerotic lesions, but neither was their definite role in the aforementioned lesions known fifteen years ago. It is with this in mind that all forms of atherosclerotic lesions will be reviewed, and where no facts have been established, some 'reasonable speculation' regarding the possible involvement of the smooth muscle cells will be attempted and areas of potential research suggested.

It has been accepted by many, although not by all, investigators in the field of atherosclerosis [120, 201] that there are three morphologically distinct forms of early atherosclerotic lesions: (1) focal intimal edema recognized in the gross as a grey gelatinous elevation, (2) microthrombi which may or may not be discernible on gross examination, and (3) focal intimal lipid accumulations recognized by the naked eye as yellow dots and streaks. These three early lesions may appear in a 'pure' form, or be a combination of any two or all three, and each may be the precursor of the advanced, clinically important, fibrous atherosclerotic plaque. Pathogenetic mechanisms that are possibly operational in the evolution from the early lesions to the advanced fibrous plaque were discussed in detail in a recent publication [120].

In the following presentation, atherosclerotic lesions will be viewed largely in the context of the role the smooth muscle cells do or may play in the inception and progression of all forms of these lesions.

Focal Intimal Edema

This lesion has been the subject of 'neglect' on the one hand and controversy on the other, as in the 'purest' form it does not contain fat in an appreciable amount; thus, it does not meet the criterion set by some investigators to qualify as an atherosclerotic lesion ('no fat, no atherosclerotic lesion'). Attention was drawn to this lesion early in this century by German pathologists [230], who observed that it was often present in the arterial intima otherwise either unaffected or accompanied by the obviously atherosclerotic (yellow) lesions; it was considered to be the lesion of inception that may or may not acquire fat, and contributes to the fibrous tissue of the atherosclerotic plaque. Renewed efforts to stress the importance of this lesion were made in Germany since the fifth decade of the century [53, 185, 240]; but acknowledgement that the lesion existed at all was extremely slow in coming on the North American continent. Initial attempts by a team of pathologists at popularizing the concept that this lesion occurs and represents a form of atherosclerotic lesions have not been entirely successful, to say the least [105, 108, 114, 190, 201]. Nevertheless, in recent years investigators have recognized that this lesion occurs, and may be produced experimentally in a variety of animal species by 'atherogenic devices' [241, 251, 252]. It has been acknowledged that focal intimal accumulations of substances derived from the lumen play an important role in the pathogenesis of atherosclerotic lesions [2, 208, 288]; the previously-stressed difference in the focal influx into versus efflux from intima as a pathogenetic factor of these intimal accumulations became popular recently [47]. Some workers purport to show that experimental hypercholesterolemic atherosclerosis may be prevented when the occurrence of the (initial) local edema is inhibited by the administration of several substances, independent of any effect on the plasma cholesterol level [253]. However, the above purported prevention has not been entirely clarified or confirmed to date.

The concept that focal intimal edema is important in atherosclerosis derives support from clinical and experimental observations that hypertension aggravates this lesion; one way by which it may affect the lesion is by an increased influx of blood constituents into the intima when overstretching of the arterial wall occurs [62, 133, 276].

Microscopically, the grey, gelatinous circumscribed elevations show intimal edema that may affect only the superficial layers or extend deep into the intima, and may reach the level of the internal elastic lamina. The edema fluid may be either purely serous or contain in addition a variable amount of fibrin that may be in the form of fine threads or clumped and conglomerated; fibrinoid is often present in the depth of a prominent lesion that shows evidence of repeated episodes of edema. The milder the lesion, i.e. the more superficial the edema that is purely serous in nature, the more inconspicuous are the changes in the intimal components: the edema fluid separates the collagen and elastic tissue fibers and the intimal smooth muscle cells, but does not necessarily alter their structure. The only intimal component that is invariably changed even in the mildest lesions is the ground substance. The change in ground substance is much better demonstrated by histochemical methods and light microscopy than by electron microscopy, because the dilution or depolymerization of acid mucopolysaccharides of the ground substance is indicated by changes in metachromasia, but can not be objectively assessed in routinely processed tissue for electron microscopy. Fragmentation, distortion and ultimate complete lysis of the extracellularly formed components of intimal connective tissue represent successive steps in progressively severe lesions; remnants of these fibers may be seen permeated or intermingled with the blood proteins contained in the edema fluid. It may also be stated that, with increased severity of the lesion, fibrin is a prominent feature in the edema, and extracellular lipids appear and may become conspicuous.

In mild lesions containing only serous edema, the smooth muscle cells in the intima may be normal. The 'fate' of these cells in the increasingly severe lesions has not been studied in detail to date. Nevertheless, by light microscopy, the gelatinous elevations show at times a variable number of fat-containing cells in addition to edema. Since we do know that most of these cells are smooth muscle cells, the intracellular fat accumulation in the largely edematous areas may be interpreted as fatty metamorphosis of smooth muscle cells, secondary (presumably) to prevailing hypoxic or other adverse local conditions that may result from the prolonged state of an unabsorbed stagnated edema fluid. The metabolic status, behavior and fate of the intimal smooth muscle cells in the grey gelatinous elevations have not been followed to date; this unknown area should provide a fruitful field for future investigations.

Mural Thrombi

Strictly speaking, one must distinguish mural thrombi that represent the initial (early) lesions of atherosclerosis from those that are involved in the growth and thus progression of an established lesion.

In the past century, VON ROKITANSKY [236] put forward the theory that atherosclerotic lesions result from the deposition of blood, notably fibrin, on the intima and from secondary degenerative changes that follow that deposition. He implied that literally all lesions begin in that fashion and that the mural deposition was a sequence to a pre-existing alteration in the coagulability of the blood, a blood 'dyscrasia'. When his abandoned theory was revived in this century [37, 59, 60, 170], it gained at first only limited support [43, 108, 110, 191], because it was difficult to reconcile with the observations and facts relevant to atherosclerosis that emerged in the meantime. Thus, it was learned that experimental hypercholesterolemia was associated with the appearance of arterial fatty dots and streaks that resembled those observed in men of all ages, and that experimental conditions could be manipulated in such a way that these fatty dots and streaks progressed to lesions similar to those of human atherosclerotic plaques. Evidence in support of the evolution of the fibrous plaque from the fatty dots and streaks accumulated, and the latter have been generally considered to represent early lesions of atherosclerosis. This being so – went the argument –, VON ROKITANSKY and his followers in this century are wrong in considering the mural thrombi to represent early lesions; moreover, it had been repeatedly pointed out that VON ROKITANSKY incorrectly ascribed the inception of lesions to a blood dyscrasia; rather, the factor important in and for the development of atherosclerotic lesions was hyperlipidemia. On the other hand, the role of mural thrombosis in the progression of lesions has been accepted in the past two decades [43, 108, 110, 191, 192, 222].

The argument that mural thrombi cannot represent early atherosclerotic lesions because fatty dots and streaks do, and that hyperlipidemia rather than changes in blood coagulability are important in atherogenesis, are no longer valid. It has been shown that organized small and large mural thrombi or thrombotic emboli induced experimentally resemble in some or most features atherosclerotic plaques [18, 98, 100, 123, 181]. Furthermore, there is evidence that a variety of lipids may promote thrombosis either through alterations in the fibrinolytic system or influencing platelets. The coagulation of blood may be enhanced by a high content of dairy fat in the diet and hyperlipemia [61, 172], phospholipids rich in phosphatidyl ethanolamine [223], and saturated long-chain fatty acids [41]. Alimentary lipemia and butter intake are alleged to inhibit fibrinolytic activity [27, 94]; diets rich in dairy fats and eggs increase the turnover and adhesiveness of platelets [205].

It is apparent that mural thrombi on the one hand and fatty dots and streaks on the other are not mutually exclusive as early atherosclerotic lesions, but represent different early forms of the lesions, and, moreover, may be interrelated through the plasma components. Nevertheless, only a modest minority strongly support the concept that mural thrombi may also represent early lesions of atherosclerosis [43, 59, 60, 108, 110, 122, 191, 192, 203, 205, 220, 221].

As early atherosclerotic lesions mural thrombi are usually small and, indeed, in most instances, may be detected only by chance on microscopic examination (fig. 5). When visible on gross examination, they are usually polypoid or 'pedunculated'. In order to 'qualify' as an early lesion, the mural thrombus must be deposited on an intima that appears normal, at least at the level examined; obviously, this is not always possible to ascertain even by ultrastructural examination. Moreover, a structurally normal intima may not necessarily be normal from a functional or biochemical point of view – but we have no means at present to assess these parameters in a very localized small intimal area. The status of the endothelium underlying the mural thrombus is even more difficult to assess, the (simplified) assumption being that it is always altered at the time of, or shortly following the deposition of thrombus.

The micromural thrombi may consist largely of either fibrin or platelets, or be mixed and have varying proportions of the two main components; they may also show trapped red blood cells. It had been suggested [12, 169] that microthrombi are being deposited at all times on normal and altered intimal surfaces, but are lysed by an effective fibrinolytic system. The observation that microthrombi may be found on the atherosclerotic and normal arterial surfaces in different animal species supports this theory [44, 70, 84].

Under pathological conditions, when the lysis does not ensue, the microthrombi become incorporated into the intimal substance by the process of organization. That microthrombi are particularly prone to occur at locations corresponding to the sites of atherosclerotic lesions has been demonstrated in experiments with extracorporeal shunts [203]. When microthrombi are rich in platelets, substances released from the latter may increase local permeability [205] resulting in focal intimal edema, as outlined in the preceding section. A microthrombus that is not lysed but becomes organized and incorporated into the intima represents a nidus for either subsequent thrombus deposition or focal edema, and may cause changes in the underlying intima [120]. Do the intimal smooth muscle cells enter the latter consideration or are they associated in yet another way with the phenomenon of deposition and outcome of microthrombi? It is conceivable that when thrombi persist and undergo organization, the metabolism and nutritional state of the intimal smooth muscle cells immediately subjacent to the thrombus is altered, and this may result in fatty metamorphosis; microthrombi of 'advanced age' (i.e., partly or entirely organized and/or hyalinized) are at times observed over an intima harboring a few fat-containing smooth muscle cells – not unlike those seen in a small fatty dot. It is, however, not always an easy task to decide whether the accumulation of fat in the smooth muscle cells preceded or followed the deposition of microthrombi; this aspect of the early atherosclerotic lesions should be studied sequentially and in detail.

Smooth muscle cells are involved in and possibly are entirely responsible for the organization of microthrombi. Over a decade ago, it was shown by light microscopy that cells concerned with the organization of large mural thrombi in human atherosclerotic lesions were smooth muscle cells rather than fibroblasts, as believed until then [108, 109, 112]. The ability of smooth muscle to organize thrombi has been demonstrated in several animal species, using different experimental models for thrombus formation [141, 142, 225]. However, no definite information is available with respect to a similar role that smooth muscle cells may play in the organization of microthrombi. Whereas the conditions of organization of tiny microthrombi over a (supposedly) normal intima are no doubt different from those prevailing in large mural thrombi often superimposed upon each other or overlying an atheroma-bearing lesion, the role of the smooth muscle cells in the latter circumstance should provide a stimulus for testing the same with respect to the former; this should prove a fruitful field for future research.

The Fatty Streak

The third form of early lesion of atherosclerosis is generally referred to as the fatty streak or fatty dot. This lesion is characterized by the presence of histochemically demonstrable lipid in the intima which may be associated with the edematous intimal lesion or mural thrombosis. The fatty streak often is referred to as a lesion exhibiting lipid deposition because of studies showing that the lipid present in the lesion in greatest amount, cholesterol, is derived primarily, if not entirely, from the blood. Summaries of studies on cholesterol influx and efflux in arteries and on lipid composition of the lesions are available for readers interested in more detailed information [47, 83]. The fact that cholesterol in the fatty streak is derived largely, if not entirely, from the blood does not mean that all lipids in the lesion are derived from the blood. Present evidence indicates that much, if not all, of the phospholipids are derived from synthesis by cells in the intima [255]. Intracellular lipid in fatty streaks also may be the result of cellular degeneration.

The typical fatty streak is a flat or slightly elevated lesion that appears as a yellow or yellow-white streak or dot in the arterial intima. The incidence and extent of intimal surface coverage of fatty streaks in various segments of the arterial vasculature and in various human populations have been well documented in an epidemiological study [85]. The term fatty streak or dot is defined by the gross appearance of the lesion. The microscopic appearance of the lesion is highly variable. In general, the lesion consists of cells with droplets of lipid in their cytoplasm and a variable amount of fine droplets or granules of lipid that appear to be in the extracellular space. The number of cells in the intima may be similar to or increased over that seen in adjacent intima in which stainable lipid is not present. The lipid-containing cells can be broadly classified into two types on the basis of cell shape. One cell type is elongated or irregularly shaped and may have few or a large number of lipid droplets in the cytoplasm. These cells are a constant component of fatty streaks, varying only in the number seen and the amount of lipid in the cells (fig. 6a). The second cell type generally is larger than the first and is ovoid in shape. The cytoplasm of this second cell type typically contains a large number of droplets of lipid of uniform size that appear to occupy the entire cytoplasm. In tissue sections where the tissue has been delipidated in processing, the second cell type shows a foamy cytoplasm representing vacuoles from which lipid has been extracted; for this reason, the cell is referred to as a 'foam cell' (fig. 6b). The large, ovoid foam cells may be numerous in a fatty streak lesion or may not be present at all. The irregularly shaped cells, with or without lipid droplets in their cytoplasm, are found throughout the thickness of the intima, i.e. superficially near the endothelium, as well as deep in the intima near the internal elastic lamina or membrane. Many of these irregularly shaped cells, as we shall discuss later, are recognizable in electron micrographs as smooth muscle; as was observed in diffuse intimal thickening, those near the internal elastic membrane or lamina are larger and better differentiated smooth muscle cells than those near the endothelium. The ovoid-shaped foam cells, when present in fatty streaks, vary in their localization in the intima, with some lesions having such cells aggregated near the endothelium, others with localization deeper in the intima, and still others with these foam cells scattered throughout the intima. The amount of lipid in fatty streaks represented by fine droplets or granules of lipid-staining material in the extracellular space is highly variable. There is no consistent relation between the amount of lipid seen extracellularly with that present intracellularly, nor is their any correlation with the type of lipid-containing cells present. Fatty streak lesions can be found that contain primarily extracellular lipid with very little intracellular lipid; such lesions have been interpreted to represent an early stage of lipid deposition [8, 11, 55, 57, 79] (fig. 4a, b). Typically, the fatty lesion, consisting largely of what appears to be extracellular lipid, is not visible in the intimal surface of an artery unless the artery has been stained with a lipid stain such as Sudan IV [78, 82].

The connective tissues found in fatty streaks are the same as those found in diffuse intimal thickening but may vary in amount. Special stains may show an apparent increase in mucopolysaccharides [23, 188], which represents a stage in the development of an edematous lesion. The internal elastic membrane or lamina may appear disrupted or frayed at the base of a fatty streak. Elastic fibers in the intima or forming a part of the internal elastic lamina may show aggregation of extracellular lipid on or about them, an appearance which has been interpreted as elastic fiber degeneration [117] (fig. 4a, b).

Identification of lipid-containing cells in fatty streaks was a subject for speculation for many years (see chapt. II) before electron microscopists showed beyond any doubt that many of the lipid-containing cells are smooth muscle [75, 111, 214]. All electron microscopic studies of both human and experimental lesions of which we are aware have confirmed the presence of lipid-containing smooth muscle cells in the lesions [88]. This finding has stimulated renewed interest in the smooth muscle cell, rediscovering its function in connective tissue formation and lipid metabolism. The cell has been referred to today as a multifunctional mesenchymal cell [86].

In the electron microscope, a number of cells can be distinguished morphologically in fatty streaks; these cells, with the exception of foam cells, are the same as those described in diffuse intimal thickening, and any or all such cells found in fatty streaks may have lipid droplets in their cytoplasm. An ovoid-shaped cell, morphologically identical to a blood monocyte, is present in fatty streaks – usually in the superficial portion of the intima near the endothelium (fig. 10, 15, 16). Also in the superficial area of the intima, there may be found irregularly shaped cells, roughly stellate (fig. 8–11). Fatty streak lesions contain smooth muscle cells, many of which have lipid inclusions in their cytoplasm (fig. 12–15, 18, 24). The structure of the smooth muscle cells in the lesion is variable and, as was observed in diffuse intimal thickening, the better differentiated cells are located near the internal elastic lamina and the less differentiated near the endothelium. For practical purposes, we can describe morphologically two types of smooth muscle cells in the lesions. Near the internal elastic lamina, the smooth muscle cells are larger than those near the endothelium and have numerous, typical myofilaments in their cytoplasm, as well as the other, but less characteristic, features of smooth muscle – numerous pinocytotic vesicles in the cell membrane and a complete limiting basement membrane (fig. 12). The smaller and less typical smooth muscle cells near the endothelium are variable in shape, generally tending to be stellate with short, thick extensions of their cytoplasm from the cell body (fig. 9–11) – in contrast to the more fusiform or strap-shape of the well-differentiated smooth muscle cells near the internal elastic lamina (fig. 12). The most noteworthy difference between the two cells is the paucity of myofilaments in the cytoplasm of the smaller cells near the endothelium. The myofilaments present in the cytoplasm usually are localized in the region of the plasma membrane and vary from the presence of a few thin filaments of questionable identity to groups of filaments with characteristic dense bodies, more readily recognizable as myofilaments. The small cells generally show an apparent increase in other organelles in the cytoplasm – mitochondria and profiles of endoplasmic reticulum (fig. 9–11). The apparent increase in some cases probably is relative, reflecting the lesser area of cytoplasm occupied by myofilaments and associated small cytoplasmic area. In other cases, there may be an absolute increase in the number of cytoplasmic organelles over that present in the larger and better differentiated smooth muscle cells. The smaller cells usually have only portions of a limiting basement membrane along the cell membrane and in some the limiting basement membrane is complete. These cells have been referred to by some as modified smooth muscle or undifferentiated cells, but usage of these terms conveys little information, as there are no rigid criteria defining them; they simply are cells that are smaller, more variable in shape, and have fewer cytoplasmic myofilaments than typical smooth muscle cells. Large, ovoid lipid-containing cells may be present in fatty streak lesions which correspond to the foam cells observed by light microscopy (fig. 21–23). Mast cells are found in small number in most human fatty streaks and are identified by their characteristic inclusions [78, 80] (fig. 23).

Endothelial cells are a constant component of fatty streaks and are identified by their anatomical location. Most electron microscopic studies of human and experimental lesions have shown the endothelium overlying the fatty streak to be modified morphologically from that overlying normal intima [16, 42, 46, 77, 79, 80, 82, 215, 265] (fig. 7). Not all investigators, however, concur in this conclusion [15, 78]. The modification or alteration of the endothelium overlying a fatty streak has been described variously as an increase in cell size, number of cytoplasmic organelles, number of mitochondria, number of profiles of smooth endoplasmic reticulum, and number of Golgi membranes. Electron-dense endothelial cytoplasmic inclusions may be present [16, 198]. One form of dense inclusion is homogeneous and is identical to the lipid inclusions found in smooth muscle cells in the intima. Such lipid inclusions are more commonly found in experimentally induced than human fatty streaks. The other form of endothelial inclusion usually is more electron-dense than the previous and, typically, has a peripheral rim of electron-dense granular material; this form of inclusion generally has been regarded as the electron microscopic counterpart of lipofuscin pigment [78, 265]. Small, electron-dense endothelial cells have been described in porcine experimental lesions that have been interpreted as evidence of endothelial cell degeneration [46]. In this same experiment, the rod-shaped bodies originally described by WEIBEL and PALADE [289] were observed to be increased over controls in pigs fed an atherogenic diet. The more complex endothelial cells in fatty streaks suggest increased metabolic activity on the part of these cells; however, the nature of this activity is yet to be determined. It has been observed that endothelium over fatty streaks incorporates more thorium from the blood than does endothelium over normal intima [58, 265]. This evidence of increased incorporation of a particle from the blood may be related to the increased influx of cholesterol into vessels with fatty streaks, which has been reported by several investigators [47]. The mechanism of lipid or lipoprotein transport across the endothelium is a major unsolved problem in atherosclerosis research.

Smooth muscle cells have been identified in human and experimentally induced fatty streaks by all investigators studying such lesions in the electron microscope [88]. In these reports, one usually finds a more complete description of the morphological characteristics of a cell that identify it as smooth muscle (myofilaments, basement membrane, pinocytotic vesicles) than of the cytoplasmic organelles and inclusions. There can be no question today that smooth muscle cells play a major role in lipid metabolism in fatty streak lesions. Detailed information on why and how these cells accumulate lipid is lacking. Possible origins for smooth muscle cells in the intima have been discussed previously (chapt. IV).

Information on the mechanism by which smooth muscle cells in fatty streaks accumulate lipid inclusions in their cytoplasm is speculation based on morphology [42, 75, 78, 82]. The lipid inclusions in smooth muscle cytoplasm usually are moderately electron-dense, homogeneous, and vary in size up to 8 μm in diameter [78] (fig. 12). The number of such inclusions varies. The inclusions may be so numerous as to impart the appearance of a foam cell (fig. 21); such cells have been termed myogenic foam cells [15] to distinguish them from the ovoid foam cells which, as we will discuss, have none of the identifying morphological features of smooth muscle. Other morphological forms of lipid inclusion have been described in smooth muscle. The central zone of a homogeneous lipid inclusion may be electron-lucid, an appearance that generally has been assumed to be due to incomplete fixative penetration and extraction by solvents during tissue processing (fig. 12, 15). The homogeneous lipid inclusions usually are ovoid in shape, with a smooth contour, but may be scalloped [15] (fig. 13, 15). A reticulated-appearing lipid inclusion is the next most common type described [75,176] (fig. 14). This inclusion has a central electron-dense homogeneous zone from which radiate electron-dense strands toward the periphery of the inclusion, an appearance resembling that of a spoked-wheel. Whether the morphological variation of lipid inclusions in smooth muscle cells is a reflection of different types of lipid or is an artefact of tissue preparation, is unknown at present. It appears more likely that the variation in morphology is due to fixation and processing, because a single section usually shows only one morphological form of inclusion and not a variation that would suggest the appearance is reflecting differing lipid composition. Myelin-like figures have been seen at the margin of lipid inclusions in smooth muscle cells [15]. Whether smooth muscle cell lipid inclusions have a limiting membrane is unknown at present. Most investigators have not seen a limiting membrane [15]. At low magnification, the inclusions may have a thin peripheral rim of increased density [180, 198] resembling a limiting membrane, but, at high magnification, a trilaminar membrane is not present. It has been suggested that the peripheral dense rim may be a condensation of phospholipid [180]. Another form of inclusion has been described in smooth muscle cell cytoplasm, with a homogeneous central portion and rather thick peripheral granular rim [78] which may be lipofuscin pigment (fig. 2).

The presence of moderately electron-dense, homogeneous lipid in cisternae of agranular endoplasmic reticulum in smooth muscle cells has been interpreted as an early stage of lipid accumulation. These cisternae appear to flow together, forming the larger lipid inclusion around which no definite membrane is visible [15, 78, 80]. The morphological appearance of lipid accumulating in smooth muscle has been interpreted to reflect lipid synthesis by the cells in the agranular endoplasmic reticulum [78]. Others believe that lipid does not necessarily accumulate in sacs of endoplasmic reticulum, as it has been observed at times free in the cytoplasm, associated with separation and degeneration of myofilaments [15]. Smooth muscle cells do not show morphological changes suggesting phagocytosis of material from the extracellular space. Lipid synthesis by the smooth muscle cell, if this is indeed what is happening, should not be interpreted necessarily to mean *de novo* synthesis; it is quite possible that the products of hydrolysis of lipids in the extracellular space are transported into the cell and then are reassembled into visible lipid. Experimental studies have shown an association of glycogen particles and lipid inclusions in smooth muscle cytoplasm [82]. The significance of this observation is unknown. Tissue culture studies now being pursued in several laboratories may be helpful in the future to resolve the problem of the mechanism of lipid accumulation and to determine whether varying morphological forms of lipid inclusion are an artefact or reflect different types of lipid.

Smooth muscle cells containing a small or moderate number of cytoplasmic lipid inclusions usually, but not invariably, show an increased number of cytoplasmic organelles over that in adjacent and similar cells free of lipid inclusions [82] (fig. 13, 15). Typically, the cell has numerous cytoplasmic myofilaments in the region of the plasma membrane, with numerous mitochondria, profiles of endoplasmic reticulum, and lipid inclusions in the central area of the cell [78, 215]. The increased number of cytoplasmic organelles seen in some lipid-containing smooth muscle cells may be related to the accumulation of lipid; if so, it is difficult to understand why all such smooth muscle cells do not show this change.

The ovoid-shaped foam cell (fig. 21–23) seen in the electron microscope has a similar appearance in human and experimental lesions. The cell does not have a basement membrane. The periphery of the cell has a variable number of microvillous cytoplasmic processes extending a short distance into the surrounding interstitial tissue. The microvillous processes are thin finger-like extensions of cytoplasm in contrast to the thick processes of smooth muscle cells. The cytoplasm of the ovoid foam cell is a maze of vacuoles, many of which consist of moderately electron-dense, homogeneous lipid similar to that in smooth muscle. The homogeneous lipid inclusions in ovoid foam cells typically are less electron-dense than those seen in adjacent smooth muscle [78, 198, 273]. In addition to homogeneous lipid inclusions, the ovoid foam cell shows a number of inclusions that are electron-lucid, the lipid apparently having been extracted during tissue processing. Cytoplasmic vacuoles also are common; they contain a variety of inclusions: electron-dense granular material similar to that in the extracellular space (fig. 22, 23); homogeneous lipid mixed with electron-dense granular material; dense bodies resembling lysosomes; and electron-lucid clefts representing some type of crystal. The mitochondria in the ovoid foam cell usually are larger than those in smooth muscle and ovoid in configuration in contrast to the elongated ones in smooth muscle. The Golgi apparatus in the ovoid foam cell is prominent. The nucleus is usually centrally placed and, typically, is either round or kidney-shaped.

The mechanism of lipid accumulation in the large foam cell is unknown. It is possible, as some have suggested, that the cell enters the intima filled with lipid (see chapt. II). Investigators have observed large foam cells penetrating the endothelium of experimental lesions [55, 79, 209, 264, 265]. The direction in which the cells are moving, from the lumen into the intima or from the intima into the lumen, is not evident in static morphological studies (fig. 19, 20). Foam cells penetrating the endothelium have been reported in only one study of human lesions [265]. We believe that present evidence strongly supports the view that foam cells are formed in the intima. The cell could accumulate lipid by a process similar to that proposed for smooth muscle cells – hydrolysis of extracellular lipids at the plasma membrane, incorporation of the products of hydrolysis into the cytoplasm, and reassembly into visible lipid. It has been suggested that these cells act as macrophages and phagocytose extracellular lipid [15, 16, 55, 77–79, 180, 265]. Inclusions are commonly observed in large foam cells containing material similar, morphologically, to that in the extracellular space; however, this resemblance is not necessarily too meaningful, as it represents one amorphous substance appearing like another (fig. 18–20, 24). It has been suggested that some of the lipid phagocytosed by the ovoid foam cell has its source in smooth muscle cells that have lost their lipid to the extracellular space [15, 112]. Lipid inclusions in ovoid foam cells differ from those in smooth muscle cells by the presence of a limiting membrane [15].

The origin of the ovoid foam cell is a subject of controversy. There are four possible cells of origin: endothelium, smooth muscle (including modified or poorly differentiated smooth muscle), blood monocytes, and interlamellar connective tissue cells. Presently available morphological data are not sufficient to resolve this controversy.

Endothelial origin of foam cells has been suggested by a number of investigators (see chapt. II). The presence of myosin-like protein and lipid droplets in the cytoplasm of endothelial cells supports this possibility and, additionally, the possibility that endothelial cells proliferating into the intima could differentiate into smooth muscle cells. In both human and experimental lesions, we have not observed morphological evidence to support an endothelial origin of intimal ovoid foam cells. Lipid inclusions in the cytoplasm of endothelial cells over human lesions are not frequently observed. Endothelial lipid inclusions are more numerous in experimental lesions, but we have not observed changes suggesting incorporation of such cells into the deeper portions of the intimal [80].

The fact that the ovoid foam cell differs morphologically from smooth muscle and that cells resembling blood monocytes are present in the lesions, with varying numbers of cytoplasmic lipid inclusions (fig. 17), has prompted the suggestion that blood monocytes enter the lesion and then accumulate lipid to become ovoid foam cells [15, 16, 77–80, 82, 180, 265]. Cells resembling monocytes are far more numerous in fatty streaks than in 'normal' intima, and what appear to be transitional stages to foam cells can be found [78, 120]. Monocytes entering a tissue are known to act as macrophages [64]; thus, the suggestion is plausible; however, more evidence than static morphology is needed to substantiate the suggestion.

We probably can state at this time that most investigators favor a smooth muscle cell origin for foam cells. That smooth muscle cells may not be the origin of ovoid foam cells was first suggested to one of us (J.C.G.) in a study of canine experimental atherosclerosis [77]. In dog lesions induced by dietary cholesterol and suppression of thyroid function, large foam cells accumulate in the intima and media (primarily media) of the vessel displacing the endothelium and musculo-elastic lamina of the media; lipid accumulation occurs in smooth muscle cells, but is infrequent, and affected cells seldom have more than two to three inclusions. In such lesions, there are small ovoid cells identical to blood monocytes that show transitional stages to the large foam cell. Similar cells are found in human lesions, and transitional stages to the large foam cell can be found [78, 120]. Such cells could be undifferentiated or unidentified resident cells of the intima, if such indeed exist (see chapt. IV). It is conceivable that such cells could proliferate in response to injury (lipid deposition) and either become ovoid foam cells or differentiate into smooth muscle. It is also possible that there are two different cells in the intima; one is similar to the interlamellar connective tissue cell, described in avian species, and the other is smooth muscle. The interlamellar connective tissue cell has been suggested as the origin of the foam cell in avian lesions [198]. If there is a counterpart of this cell in mammalian species, it could be the progenitor of the ovoid foam cell. We cannot resolve this problem on the basis of current information. The basic question is whether the cell in the intima resembling a blood monocyte is a blood monocyte or is a resident cell of the intima that, in mammalian species, is normally present in small number.

The fact that the ovoid foam cell has none of the morphological features that identify smooth muscle in an electron micrograph does not necessarily exclude smooth muscle as the cell of origin. It is possible that the smooth muscle cell, as it accumulates lipid, loses its myofilaments, basement membrane, and pinocytotic vesicles. We cannot deny this possibility, but it seems unlikely, as we see large myogenic foam cells that retain the identifying characteristics of smooth muscle (fig. 21). The less well differentiated smooth muscle cells found in diffuse intimal thickening and fatty streaks near the endothelium represent another possible cell of origin for ovoid foam cells. These cells, often referred to as modified smooth muscle, and their possible origin in the intima were discussed in chapter IV. We believe these cells are not likely to be the origin of ovoid foam cells, because we have observed such cells to contain lipid inclusions less often than do the typical or well-differentiated smooth muscle cells. BALIS *et al.* [16] have made a similar observation in experimental lesions. These cells thus do not appear to have a great tendency for accumulating cytoplasmic lipid inclusions. The poorly differentiated or modified smooth muscle cells often have cytoplasmic cisternae of granular endoplasmic reticulum; it is possible that their function is connective tissue elaboration rather than lipid accumulation.

Droplets or granules staining positively for lipid in the extracellular space in fatty streaks have been noted consistently by light microscopists. On the basis of correlated light and electron microscopic studies, it has been concluded that the electron microscopic counterpart of the extracellular stainable lipid seen by light microscopy are electron-dense particles of highly variable appearance in the interstitial space [77, 80, 82]. The interstitial particles vary in electron density from moderate to marked and are variable in size and shape (fig. 7, 9, 10, 12–17, 21, 24). Some of the particles have a laminated (myelin-like) appearance [180]. Numerous investigators have observed these dense interstitial particles in both human and experimental lesions [15, 32, 76–80, 82, 117, 180, 198, 215, 260, 265, 273]. We probably are safe in stating that all fatty streak lesions contain the dense interstitial particles; the amount varies. Despite the prominence of interstitial dense particles in lesions, they have not been discussed often with regard to their identity and source [15, 16, 76, 77, 80, 82, 117, 198]. All reports agree that these particles contain lipid as at least one of their components. The source of these particles has never been conclusively demonstrated; however, several possible sources have been suggested. These possible sources include degeneration of elastic fibers [117], degeneration of lipid-containing smooth muscle cells [15], precipitated blood lipoprotein [77, 78, 82], degeneration of foam cells [82, 209, 264], or all of these [117]. The most likely sources appear to be cell degeneration or lipoprotein derived from the blood that has precipitated in the extracellular space. These two possible sources are not mutually exclusive.

Connective tissue structures in the interstitial space of fatty streaks are the same as those observed in diffuse intimal thickening – collagen, elastic fibers, basement membranes, and microfibrils. Elastic fibers, especially those comprising the internal elastic lamina, may show aggregation of the interstitial electron-dense particles around them, which probably represents the electron microscopic counterpart of the lipid encrustation of elastic fibers observed by light microscopy [78]. Fibrin has been identified in the interstitial tissue of fatty streaks [114, 117], which may indicate a previous mural thrombus or reflect an increase in endothelial permeability.

Mast cells have been found in fatty streaks in small number [78]. The mast cells may show lipid inclusions in their cytoplasm which, typically, are few in number and more electron-dense than those seen in smooth muscle cells (fig. 23). Mast cells are found in human fatty streaks consistently, although in small number, which suggests that they play some role in the formation or regression of the lesion. Mast cells in human lesions are readily identified by their characteristic cytoplasmic inclusions, vacuoles containing cylindrical, electron-dense bodies that, at high magnification, have a laminated structure (fig. 23).

The morphological stages in the development of a fatty streak cannot be described with certainty for any species, because we cannot observe the changes sequentially at a given site in the vasculature of a single animal. We must rely on duration of cholesterol feeding, degree and duration of hyperlipemia, amount of lipid in the lesion, or age of the subject (human) to surmise whether the changes observed are early or late in the development of the lesion. Further, it is clearly evident in experimental models that all fatty streak lesions do not begin their development at the same time and achieve the same size or lipid content. In any given animal or man, fatty streak lesions of varying size, lipid content and cellular composition can be found. This observation indicates that either the lesions begin their development at different times or evolve at different rates. Although there is no way known at present to differentiate between these two possibilities, it seems likely that both obtain – lesions begin to develop at various times depending on the local factors that permit lipid deposition, and also evolve at different rates, which is likewise a function of local factors. This conclusion emphasizes local factors as being of prime importance both in the inception and progression of a lesion. Fatty streak lesions can be induced in animals by any manipulation that results in a marked and sustained increase in circulating beta-lipoproteins (cholesterol-rich lipoproteins). If the vasculature acted as an inert filter, we should expect to see rather generalized lipid deposition, proportionate to the hyperlipemia influenced to some degree by pressure and flow characteristics. We do not see a generalized deposition of lipid in the vasculature. There are specific segments of the vasculature that characteristically develop the lesions, and these segments vary between species. Thus, there can be no question that local factors are of prime importance in the inception and progression of lesions. The unsolved problem, which is a subject of diverse opinion, is the nature and relative importance of various local factors in the inception and progression of a lesion.

If we can accept that local factors are of prime importance in the inception and progression of a lesion, we must next better define these factors. The basic question is: Why are blood lipids deposited in the arterial intima? What is the role of endothelial permeability? Do changes in vascular connective tissues facilitate or cause lipid deposition? Are there changes in intimal cell functions that result in lipid accumulation or alteration in intimal connective tissues? Does intimal thickening facilitate lipid deposition? What is the role of hemodynamic factors in altering endothelial permeability and stimulating changes in intimal cells and connective tissue composition? Quite obviously, all the above are interrelated and probably have relative roles in the phenomenon of lipid deposition. What we do not know is: which are the more important, and is there one that begins the process resulting in a cascade-type reaction? Presently we are rather limited in our ability to decipher this puzzle. The limitation of not being able to observe either functionally or morphologically the evolution of one lesion in one animal has led to various interpretations and controversy. Further, our major investigative tool has been, and still largely is, morphology. It is not necessary that all functional changes be reflected in morphological changes, even when observed at the level of the electron microscope. Thus, there may well be key functional changes that occur in intimal cells and connective tissues prior to lipid deposition, that eventually facilitate or cause lipid deposition. We are searching for the 'initial lesion' that represents a functional change in the intima that may or may not have a morphological reflection. Two possible morphological forms for the 'initial lesion' have been discussed in this section, the edematous lesion and mural thrombosis, but we recognize that these morphological manifestations may be the end result of functional changes in the cells and connective tissues of the intima. For example, an alteration in endothelial cell surface characteristics induced by hemodynamic stresses could result in platelet deposition and thrombosis (morphologic) which, in turn, results in increased endothelial permeability (functional). The passage of increased amounts of plasma into the intima could result in intimal swelling (morphologic) and induction of changes in intimal cell function (may have morphologic reflection). The greater resolution of morphological changes by the electron microscope has shown clearly that smooth muscle cell number and structure are modified in fatty streaks, but has not clarified the sequence of changes that occur with inception and progression of the lesions.

The presence of stainable lipid in a lesion provides us with an easily recognizable morphological marker for studying lesion progression. Considering the lesion only from the time that lipid deposition can be observed, there is experimental evidence that the earliest lesion of lipid deposition is the presence of lipid-staining droplets or granules in the interstitial space [8, 11, 55, 57]. The next morphological stage in fatty streak development is the appearance of intracellular stainable lipid. The intracellular lipid may be derived in part from cellular degeneration, but it would appear from flux studies that most of the cholesterol, the predominant lipid component, is derived from the blood plasma. However, some investigators have shown evidence that lipid may appear first in the cells, the extracellular lipids not exceeding the amount observed in normal intimas [120].

Fatty streaks are considered by most students of the lesions to be reversible, though the evidence for this is meager. Experimental studies of lesion regression are few in number. ANITSCHKOW [8] observed that when hypercholesterolemic rabbits were returned to a normal diet, the lesions showed a diminution in the number of foam cells, the appearance of an extracellular mass of lipid debris (atheromatous core), the appearance of elongated cells beneath the endothelium associated with collagen and elastic fibers, and modification of the shape of smooth muscle cells in the media subjacent to the atheromatous core. It is difficult to consider the lesion observed as representing reversal or regression. Histologically, the lesion has assumed the appearance of an atheromatous plaque and thus indicates progression. More recently, regression has been studied in rhesus monkeys [9]. Judging from the light micrographs included in the publication, during the period the monkeys were on a diet without added cholesterol, there was a marked decrease in the amount of lipid in the lesions, resulting in fibromuscular intimal plaques of considerably less volume than the lesions observed at the end of the period of feeding a diet with added cholesterol. The lesions at the end of the feeding period resembled diffuse intimal thickening observed in human arteries (see chapt. IV). The regression lesions described in these two species differ with regard to the appearance of an atheromatous core. The reason for this difference is unknown, but could be related to the amount of lipid initially present or the cellular response to lipid in the two species. The common feature of these two species during the period of lesion regression appears to be the loss of large foam cells from the lesions. Passage of arterial lipid to adventitial lymphatics may occur in canine experimental lesions [25], but we are unaware of evidence for this movement in other species. Another mechanism by which the number of foam cells in lesions may be reduced is necrosis of the cells and release of the lipid into the extracellular space. The electron-dense cytoplasmic inclusions in foam cells containing material morphologically similar to the extracellular lipid-containing material has been interpreted as evidence for phagocytosis [77–79]; however, a cell with such inclusions often shows evidence of cellular degeneration – nuclear chromatin clumping, mitochondrial swelling, and disruption of the plasma membrane [16, 80]. Such electron-dense cytoplasmic inclusions may well represent cytoplasmic degeneration. Necrosis of foam cells was previously discussed as a possible origin for the extracellular electron-dense, lipid-containing material [82, 120, 209, 264]. Cellular necrosis obviously could result in the atheromatous core ANITSCHKOW observed in rabbit lesions. In the rhesus monkey, it is possible that fewer foam cells are present in the fatty streaks at the end of the period a diet with added cholesterol was fed, or they more readily exit the vessel or both. We can only speculate on the possibilities. Foam cells in experimental lesions typically are located immediately beneath the endothelium [180, 273] and thus do not have far to travel to exit the vessel (fig. 19, 20). Morphological changes indicative of degeneration or necrosis have also been described in smooth muscle cells [15, 46, 75]. Smooth muscle cell necrosis may play a role in fatty streak regression or progression to development of a plaque. Morphological changes reflecting regression or progression of human fatty streaks are entirely unknown. Detailed morphological studies of the development and regression of experimental fatty streaks including electron microscopy should be very valuable in furthering our understanding of the cellular reactions that occur during lipid deposition and the fate of the deposited lipid.

Fatty streaks do not by themselves cause disease. Our interest in the fatty streak is based on the assumption that some of these lesions progress to become fibrous plaques or atheromatous plaques which have the potential for causing disease. The role of the fatty streak in the evolution of plaques is a subject of controversy, with some believing they have no role. For this presentation, we are assuming that some fatty streaks remain static, some regress, and still others progress to fibrous plaques. The mechanism by which a fatty streak transforms to a fibrous plaque is not known. It has been suggested that cellular necrosis and connective tissue damage in the intima are some of the stimuli for deposition of fibrous connective tissue and plaque formation [80, 120]. Sclerogenic properties of lipids have been studied and support this suggestion [1]. Morphological evidence of cell necrosis has been described in fatty streaks, as discussed previously. Necrosis of lipid-containing cells forming an atheromatous core and stimulating fibrous tissue formation could be a mechanism for transforming a fatty streak into a plaque. It is also possible that fatty streaks have no or very little role in plaque formation. Perhaps whatever it is that generates a plaque may do so in an area where fatty streaks are caught up in the process.

VI. The Fibrous Plaque

The term fibrous plaque, like that of the fatty streak, refers to the gross appearance of the lesion and does not imply any particular or constant histological picture. The fibrous plaque is a firm, gray-white, mound-like lesion in the arterial intima that varies in size from a few millimeters to over one centimeter. The lesion, when sectioned through its central portion, typically contains a variable amount of gruel-like material that represents the 'atheroma', which is composed of extracellular lipid rich in cholesterol. The incidence and extent of fibrous plaques in the human vasculature has been well documented [85].

The structures observed in fibrous plaques by light microscopy are more variable than those in fatty streaks. The small and less complex fibrous plaques observed in the third and fourth decades of life perhaps are the early stage of evolution of the highly complex or complicated lesions seen later in life. The typical uncomplicated fibrous plaque is composed of a core of extracellular lipid debris, exhibiting a variable number of crystals of cholesterol and an overlying layer or cap of collagen and thin, elongated cells. The core or atheroma is near the media; the fibro-cellular cap covers the core on the luminal side of the lesion like a blanket isolating a noxious substance from direct view (fig. 25). The fibro-cellular cap is covered by endothelium. The amount of lipid comprising the atheromatous core varies from massive relative to the volume of the lesion, to so small an amount as to raise the question of the primacy of lipid in the evolution of the lesion. A possible pathogenesis for the formation of fibrous plaques was discussed previously – necrosis of cells in fatty streaks releasing lipid into the extracellular space serving as a stimulus to reactive fibrosis. Another possible pathogenesis for the uncomplicated fibrous plaque is successive deposition and organization of mural thrombi. These two possible mechanisms for plaque formation are not mutually exclusive and do not preclude the possibility of yet other mechanisms being operative. The primary stimulus to and pathogenesis of fibrous plaque formation unquestionably represent the most important areas for future research, if we are to prevent or control the diseases caused by atherosclerosis.

With time, the uncomplicated fibrous plaque may undergo a variety of morphological changes that vary from one lesion to another. These changes generally are referred to as complications and the resulting lesion as a complicated fibrous plaque. Vascularization is a common change in fibrous plaques. Capillary-size vessels are seen in varying number at the periphery of the atheroma that appear to arise from adventitial vasa vasorum. Some vessels also appear to arise from the arterial lumen and are referred to as high-pressure capillaries. Associated with vascularization of the plaque, it is common to find hemorrhages into the lesion that vary in size from minuscule to massive, which undoubtedly represent one mechanism by which a fibrous plaque can increase in mass. Mural thrombosis over a plaque also is a common finding as is the presence of layers of fibrin in the fibro-cellular cap of the lesion in varying stages of organization. Thus, repeated episodes of mural thrombosis also are a mechanism by which fibrous plaques can increase in mass. Foci of calcification are commonly found in complicated fibrous plaques that appear to represent dystrophic calcification. The number and type of cells seen in and around fibrous plaques is highly variable. Foam cells may be numerous in the fibro-cellular cap or around the atheroma, and such cells may be entirely absent. Occasionally, complicated fibrous plaques are seen densely infiltrated with polymorphonuclear leukocytes. An area of coagulation necrosis is sometimes seen in the fibro-cellular cap that has the appearance of an infarction. Large numbers of lymphocytes are commonly observed in the adventitia of an artery adjacent to an area containing one or more complicated fibrous plaques. The complex morphology of complicated fibrous plaques has been studied in detail by MORGAN [196]. The cause and relative importance of these changes for plaque growth and thus clinical disease remains largely unknown. The causes for plaque growth represent another area for research that potentially could result in measures for the control or prevention of disease due to atherosclerosis.

There are few experimental models for fibrous plaques. Probably the most valid ones available at present are birds [199, 260].

There have been few electron microscopic studies of fibrous plaques. The findings of such studies, however, have been in accord as to the types of cells and connective tissue present. The cells in the fibro-cellular cap of the lesion are primarily smooth muscle recognizable by the features previously described [42, 88, 116, 119, 121, 176, 198, 199, 260]. The smooth muscle cells in the fibro-cellular cap differ morphologically from the typical smooth muscle cells in vascular media, both in shape and cytoplasmic organelles. The smooth muscle cells in the cap of a fibrous plaque are very elongated and slender, with few cytoplasmic projections extending from the cell body into the surrounding connective tissue space. The cells are oriented in the long axis of the vessel and vary in number, with some lesions having rather densely packed cells and yet others having few cells in a rather dense collagenous stroma. The cytoplasm of the smooth muscle cells contains few myofilaments and these are located primarily in the region of the plasma membrane. The central portion of the cytoplasm exhibits numerous profiles of endoplasmic reticulum, especially the granular form. Micropinocytotic vesicles are fewer in number in the plasma membrane than is observed in medial smooth muscle cells. The smooth muscle cells in the fibrous plaque usually have a complete limiting basement membrane which, in some lesions, is extremely thick (fig. 26). Lipid inclusions have been described in the cytoplasm of smooth muscle cells in plaques that are morphologically identical to those in smooth muscle cells in fatty streaks [88].

Adjacent to the endothelium, unidentified cells have been described [198, 199] that are similar to those found in diffuse intimal thickening and fatty streaks. Fibroblasts have been reported to be present in fibrous plaques [88, 176]; but distinguishing a fibroblast from the unidentified cells or modified smooth muscle is difficult and leaves serious question as to whether fibroblasts are present at all. Experimental studies of the organization of thrombi have shown smooth muscle cells to be the ones associated with the appearance of collagen [68, 204, 210, 225, 267]. Possible origins for the smooth muscle cells in the fibrous cap of a plaque are the same as those posed in discussing intimal thickening and the fatty streak (see chapt. IV, V).

Ovoid foam cells may be found in the cap of a fibrous plaque [88, 176, 198] and differ in no recognizable way from those in fatty streaks. The origin of such cells in a plaque is no more clear than it was in fatty streaks. It has been noted that spontaneous plaques in chickens change their appearance when the chickens are fed a diet with added cholesterol, with smooth muscle cells becoming vacuolated and the number of non-smooth muscle cells increasing greatly [198]. The foam cells in the lesions were not felt to arise from smooth muscle cells but rather from the non-smooth muscle interlamellar connective tissue cells [198]. As was discussed previously, we do not know whether this cell is unique to avian species or has not as yet been recognized in mammalian species.

The interstitial tissue of the fibrous cap of a plaque contains abundant collagen. Elastic fibers are few in number and are small. Basement membrane material is variable in amount and does not always appear to be associated with a cell. Interstitial electron-dense material (lipid) and fibrin also may be found [176]. There can be no question today that the cell responsible for the elaboration of connective tissues is the smooth muscle cell. The questions that remain are: Which is the stimulus to this cell that causes it to elaborate connective tissues? What is the origin of this cell? What causes it to cease elaborating connective tissues?

The extracellular atheromatous debris in the core of the fibrous plaque is composed of a large amount of electron-dense granular material [176] identical to that observed in the interstitial tissue of fatty streaks and the fibrous cap of the plaque. Among the electron-dense granular particles are electron-lucid clefts representing cholesterol crystals [176] (fig. 27). Electron-dense crystals have been described that are interpreted to be calcium-containing [75].

Electron microscopy has enabled us to identify the cell in the fibrous cap of human fibrous plaques that is responsible for connective tissue elaboration. The smooth muscle cell, at all possible stages of the evolution of an atheromatous lesion, is present, is modified morphologically from smooth muscle cells in the media, and is the predominant cell type in most human lesions. The importance of this cell in the reactions of the artery wall that eventuate in atheromatous lesions is obviously great. What remains is to determine all functional characteristics of this cell and the controlling mechanisms.

VII. Epilogue

We have decided not to follow the conventional way in which monographs, in analogy to original publications, usually are closed and we shall refrain from writing a summary or conclusions. This decision was made in view of the fact that most of the chapters and sections included closing remarks, attempting either to summarize briefly the present status pertaining to the specific subject discussed or suggesting areas for future investigations; interested readers may find these conveniently in appropriate sections.

VIII. References

1 Abdulla, Y. H.; Adams, C. W. M., and Morgan, R. S.: The reaction of connective tissues to implantation of purified sterol, sterol esters, phosphoglycerides, glycerides and free fatty acids. J. Path. Bact. *94:* 63–71 (1967).

2 Adams, C. W. M.: Atheroma lipids. J. Atheroscler. Res. *7:* 117–119 (1967).

3 Albert, Z.: Die Veränderungen der Aorta bei Kindern und ihr Verhältnis zur Atherosklerose. Virchows Arch. path. Anat. *303:* 265–279 (1939).

4 Altschul, R.: Histologic analysis of arteriosclerosis. Arch. Path *38:* 305–312 (1944).

5 Altschul, R.: Selected studies on arteriosclerosis (Thomas, Springfield 1950).

6 Altschul, R.: Endothelium (Macmillan, New York 1954).

7 Anitschkow, N. N.: A history of experimentation on arterial atherosclerosis in animals; in Blumenthal Cowdry's arteriosclerosis; 2nd ed., pp. 21–44 (Thomas, Springfield 1967).

8 Anitschkow, N.: Experimental arteriosclerosis in animals; in Cowdry Arteriosclerosis, a survey of the problem, pp. 271–322 (Macmillan, New York 1933).

9 Armstrong, M. L.; Warner, E. D., and Connor, W. E.: Regression of coronary atheromatosis in rhesus monkeys. Circulat. Res. *27:* 59–67 (1970).

10 Aschoff, L.: Lectures in pathology, p. 17 (Hoeber, New York 1924).

11 Aschoff, L.: Atherosclerosis; in Lectures on pathology, pp. 131–153 (Hoeber, New York 1924).

12 Astrup, T.: Role of blood coagulation and fibrinolysis in the pathogenesis of arteriosclerosis; in Page Connective tissue, thrombosis, and atherosclerosis, pp. 223–237 (Academic Press, New York 1959).

13 Bader, H.: The anatomy and physiology of the vascular wall; in Hamilton Handbook of physiology II. Vol. 2: Circulation, pp. 865–889 (Amer. Physiol. Soc., Washington, D.C. 1963).

14 Bailey, C. H.: Atheroma and other lesions produced in rabbits by cholesterol feeding. J. exp. Med. *23:* 69–85 (1916).

15 Balis, J. U.; Haust, M. D., and More, R. H.: Electron-microscopic studies in human atherosclerosis, cellular elements in aortic fatty streaks. Exp. molec. Path. *3:* 511–525 (1964).

16 Balis, J. U.; Chan A. S., and Conen, P. E.: The effect of postlathyritic medial scar on the progression of experimental atherosclerosis in rats. Exp. molec. Path. *8:* 90–111 (1968).

17 Barbolini, G.; Scilabra, G. A.; Botticelli, A., and Botticelli, S.: On the origin of foam cells in cholesterol-induced atherosclerosis of the rabbit. Virchows Arch. Abt. B Zellpath. *3:* 24–32 (1969).

18 BARNARD P. J.: Experimental fibrin thrombo-embolism of the lungs. J. Path. Bact. *65:* 129–136 (1953).

19 BAUM und THIENEL: Über Besonderheiten im Bau der Blutgefässe. Arch. mikroskop. Anat. *63:* 10–34 (1904).

20 BECKER, C. G. and MURPHY, G. E.: Demonstration of contractile protein in endothelium and cells of the heart valves, endocardium, intima, arteriosclerotic plaques, and Aschoff bodies of rheumatic heart disease. Amer. J. Path. *55:* 1–37 (1969).

21 BENNINGHOFF, A.: Über die Beziehungen zwischen elastischem Gerüst und glatter Muskulatur in der Arterienwand und ihre funktionelle Bedeutung. Z. Zellforsch. mikroskop. Anat. *6:* 348–396 (1928).

22 BENNINGHOFF, A.: Blutgefässe und Herz; in Handbuch der mikroskopischen Anatomie des Menschen. I, vol. 6 (Springer, Berlin 1930).

23 BERTELSEN, S.: The role of ground substance, collagen, and elastic fibers in the genesis of artherosclerosis; in SANDLER and BOURNE Atherosclerosis and its origin, pp. 119–161 (Academic Press, New York 1963).

24 BETTEX-GALLAND, M. and LUSCHER, E. F.: Thrombosthenin – a contractile protein from thrombocytes: its extraction from human blood platelets and some of its properties. Biochim. Biophys. Acta *49:* 536–547 (1961).

25 BEVANS, M.; DAVIDSON, J. D., and KENDALL, F. E.: Regression of lesions in canine arteriosclerosis. Arch. Path. *51:* 288–292 (1951).

26 BIERRING, F. and KOBAYASI, T.: Electron microscopy of the normal rabbit aorta. Acta path. microbiol. scand. *57:* 154–168 (1963).

27 BILLIMORIA, J. D.; DRYSDALE, J.; JAMES, D. C. O., and MACLAGAN, N. F.: Determination of fibrinolytic activity of whole blood with special reference to the effects of exercise and fat feeding. Lancet *ii:* 471–475 (1959).

28 BIOZZI, G.; MENE, G. et OVARY, Z.: L'histamine et la granulopexie de l'endothelium vasculaire. Rev. Immunol. *12:* 320–334 (1948).

29 BOUISSOU, H.; SENDRAIL-PESQUE, M.; JULIAN, M.; FABRE, M. T.; RUMEAU, J. L. et DURROUX, R.: La structure artérielle chez l'enfant et l'adulte jeune. Ses variations topographiques et physiologiques, ses perturbations au cours de quelques états pathologiques; dans Le rôle de la paroi artérielle dans l'athérogénèse. Coll. Int., C.N.R.S., Paris, No. 169, pp. 33–74 (1968).

30 BORK, K.: Über Kranzadersklerose. Virchows Arch. path. Anat. *262:* 646–657 (1926).

31 BREMER, J. L.: On the variations of wall thickness in embryonic arteries. Anat. Rec. *27:* 1–13 (1924).

32 BUCK, R. C.: Lesions in the rabbit aorta produced by feeding a high cholesterol diet followed by a normal diet, an electron microscopic study. Brit. J. exp. Path. *43:* 236–240 (1962).

33 BURROWS, M. T.: The cultivation of tissues of the chick embryo outside the body. J. amer. med. Ass. *55:* 2057–2058 (1910).

34 CAESAR, R.; EDWARDS, G. A., and RUSKA, H.: Architecture and nerve supply of mammalian smooth muscle tissue. J. biophys. biochem. Cytol. *3:* 867–878 (1957).

35 CASARINI, A.: Osservazioni sulle alterazioni dell intima coronarica presenti alla nascita. Biol. *3:* 68–84 (1950).

36 CHANDLER, A. B. and HAND, R. A.: Phagocytized platelets: a source of lipids in human thrombi and atherosclerotic plaques. Science *134:* 946–947 (1961).

37 Clark, E.; Graef, I., and Chasis, H.: Thrombosis of the aorta and coronary arteries with special reference to the 'fibrinoid lesions. Arch. Path. *22:* 183–212 (1936).

38 Clarkson, T. B. and Lofland, H. B.: Effects of cholesterol-fat diets on pigeons susceptible and resistant to atherosclerosis. Circulat. Res. *9:* 106 (1961).

39 Cliff, W. J.: The aortic tunica media in growing rats studied with the electron microscope. Lab. Invest. *17:* 599–615 (1967).

40 Cliff, W. J.: The aortic tunica media in aging rats. Exp. molec. Path. *13:* 172–189 (1970).

41 Connor, W. E. and Poole, J. C.: The effect of fatty acids on the formation of thrombi. Quart. J. exp. Physiol. *46:* 1–7 (1961).

42 Cooke, P. H. and Smith, S. C.: Smooth muscle cells: the source of foam cells in atherosclerotic white carneau pigeons. Exp. molec. Path. *8:* 171–189 (1968).

43 Crawford, T. and Levene, C. I.: The incorporation of fibrin in the aortic intima. J. Path. Bact. *64:* 523–528 (1952).

44 Dahme, E. G.: Atherosclerosis and arteriosclerosis in domestic animals. Ann. N.Y. Acad. Sci. *127:* 657–670 (1965).

45 Daoud, A.; Jarmolych, J.; Zumbo, A., and Fani, K.: 'Preatheroma phase of coronary atherosclerosis in man. Exp. molec. Path. *3:* 475–484 (1964).

46 Daoud, A. S.; Jones, R. and Scott, R. F.: Dietary-induced atherosclerosis in miniature swine. II. Electron microsopy observations: characteristics of endothelial and smooth muscle cells in the proliferative lesions and elsewhere in the aorta. Exp. molec. Path. *8:* 263–301 (1968).

47 Dayton, S. and Hashimoto, S.: Recent advances in molecular pathology: a review. Cholesterol flux and metabolism in arterial tissue and in atheromata. Exp. molec. Path. *13:* 253–268 (1970).

48 DeBakey, M. E.; Jordan, G. L.; Abbott, J. P.; Halpert, B., and O Neal, R. M.: The fate of dacron vascular grafts. Arch. Surg., Chicago *89:* 757–782 (1964).

49 Dewey, M. M. and Barr, L.: Intercellular connection between smooth muscle cells: the nexus. Science *137:* 670–672 (1962).

50 Dibble, J. H.: The aging and collateral peripheral artery. Lancet *i:* 520–523 (1964).

51 Dietrich, A.: Reaktive Thrombose im Tierversuch. Virchows Arch. path. Anat. *307:* 281–296 (1941).

52 Dock, W.: The predilection of atherosclerosis for the coronary arteries. J. amer. med. Ass. *131:* 875–878 (1931).

53 Doerr, W.: Perfusiontheorie der Arteriosklerose; in Bargmann und Doerr Zwanglose Abhandlungen aus dem Gebiet der normalen und pathologischen Anatomie, Heft 13 (Thieme, Stuttgart 1963).

54 Doerr, W.: Allgemeine Pathologie der Organe des Kreislaufes; in Altmann und Büchner *et al.* Handbuch der allgemeinen Pathologie. IV, vol. 3, pp. 326–327 (Springer, Berlin 1970).

55 Duff G. L.: Experimental cholesterol arteriosclerosis and its relationship to human arteriosclerosis. Arch. Path. *20:* 81–123, 259–304 (1935).

56 Duff, G.: Atherosclerosis. Canad. med. Ass. J. *64:* 387–394 (1951).

57 Duff, G. L. and McMillan G. C.: Pathology of atherosclerosis. Amer. J. Med. *11:* 92 (1951).

58 Duff G.; McMillan G. C. and Lautsch E. V.: The uptake of colloidal thorium dioxide by the arterial lesions of cholesterol atherosclerosis in the rabbit. Amer. J. Path. *30:* 941–955 (1954).

59 Duguid J. B.: Thrombosis as a factor in the pathogenesis of coronary atherosclerosis. J. Path. Bact. *58:* 207–212 (1946).

60 Duguid, J. B.: Pathogenesis of arteriosclerosis. Lancet *ii:* 925–927 (1949).

61 Duncan, G. G. and Waldron, J. M.: The effect of ingested fat on blood coagulation. Trans. Ass. amer. Physicians *62:* 179–185 (1949).

62 Duncan, L. E., jr.: Mechanical factors in the localization of atheroma; in Jones Evolution of the atherosclerotic plaque, pp. 171–182 (University of Chicago Press, Chicago 1963).

63 Easterly, J. A.; Glagov, S., and Ferguson, D. J.: Morphogenesis of intimal obliterative hyperplasia of small arteries in experimental pulmonary hypertension. Amer. J. Path. *52:* 325–347 (1968).

64 Ebert, R. H. and Florey, H. W.: The extravascular development of the monocyte observed *in vivo*. Brit. J. exp. Path. *20:* 342–356 (1939).

65 Edholm, G.: Über die Arteria Coronaria Cordis des Menschen. Anat. Anz. *42:* 124–128 (1912).

66 Ehrich, W.; Dela Chapelle, C., and Cohn, A. E.: Anatomical ontogeny; B. Man. I. A study of the coronary arteries. Amer. J. Anat. *49:* 241–282 (1931/1932).

67 Fangman, R. J. and Hellwig, C. A.: Histology of coronary arteries in newborn infants. Abstract. Amer. J. Path. *23:* 901–902 (1947).

68 Florey, H. W.; Greer, S. J.; Poole, J. C. F., and Werthessen, N. T.: The pseudointima lining fabric grafts of the aorta. Brit. J. exp. Path. *42:* 236–246 (1961).

69 French, J. E.; Jennings, M. A.; Poole, J. C. F.; Robinson, D. S., and Florey, H. W.: Intimal changes in the arteries of aging swine. Proc. roy. Soc. Med. *158:* 24–42 (1963).

70 French, J. E.; Jennings, M. A., and Florey, H. W.: Morphological studies on atherosclerosis in swine. Ann. N. Y. Acad. Sci. *127:* 780–797 (1965).

71 French, J. E.: Vascular factors and thrombosis; in Brinkhous Transactions of the conference held under the Auspices of the International Committee on Haemostasis and Thrombosis, Bath 1969; pp. 11–22 (Schattauer, Stuttgart 1970).

72 Fritz, K. E.; Jarmolych, J., and Dauod, A. S.: Association of DNA synthesis and apparent dedifferentiation of aortic smooth muscle cells *in vitro*. Exp. molec. Path. *12:* 354–362 (1970).

73 Gardiol, D.: Aspects histologiques et histochimiques de la sénescene des artères de gros et moyen calibre. Ann. Anat. path. *9:* 269–282 (1964).

74 Geer, J. C.; McGill, H. C., jr.; Strong, J. P., and Holman, R. L : Electron microscopy of human atherosclerotic lesions. Abstract. Fed. Proc. *19:* 15 (1960).

75 Geer, J. C.; McGill, H. C., and Strong, J. P.: The fine structure of human atherosclerotic lesions. Amer. J. Path. *38:* 263–287 (1961).

76 Geer, J. C. and Guidry, M. A.: Cholesteryl ester composition and morphology of human normal intima and fatty streaks. Exp. molec. Path. *3:* 485–499 (1964)

77 Geer, J. C.: Fine structure of canine experimental atherosclerosis. Amer. J. Path. *47:* 241–269 (1965).

78 Geer, J. C.: Fine structure of human aortic intimal thickening and fatty streaks. Lab. Invest. *14:* 1764–1783 (1965).

79 GEER, J. C.: Fine structure of experimental atherosclerosis; in MILLIKAN, SIEKERT and WHISNANT Cerebral vascular diseases, pp. 37–52 (Grune & Stratton, New York 1966).
80 GEER, J. C. and MCGILL, H. C., jr.: The evolution of the fatty streak; in BREST and MOYER Atherosclerotic vascular disease, pp. 8–22 (Appleton-Century-Crofts, New York 1967).
81 GEER, J. C.; MCGILL, H. C., jr.; ROBERTSON, W. B., and STRONG, J. P.: Histologic characteristics of coronary artery fatty streaks. Lab. Invest. *18:* 565–570 (1968).
82 GEER, J. C.; CATSULIS, C.; MCGILL, H. C., jr., and STRONG, J. P.: Fine structure of the baboon aortic fatty streak. Amer. J. Path. *52:* 265–285 (1968).
83 GEER, J. C.; PANGANAMALA, R. V.; NEWMAN, H. A.I., and CORNWELL, D. G.: Mural metabolism; in JONES Atherosclerosis, pp. 6–12 (Springer, New York 1970).
84 GEISSINGER, H. D.; MUSTARD, J. F., and ROWSELL, H. C.: The occurrence of microthrombi on the aortic endothelium of swine. Canad. med. Ass. J. *87:* 405–408 (1962).
85 MCGILL, H. C., jr. (ed.): Geographic pathology of atherosclerosis, pp. 653 (Williams & Wilkins, Baltimore 1968).
86 GETZ, G. S.; VESSELINOVITCH, D., and WISSLER, R. W.: A dynamic pathology of atherosclerosis. Amer. J. Med. *46:* 657–673 (1969).
87 GHANI, A. R. and TIBBS, D. J.: Role of blood-borne cells in organization of mural thrombi. Brit. med. J. *i:* 1244–1247 (1962).
88 GHIDONI, J. J. and O'NEAL, R. M.: Recent advances in molecular pathology. A review: ultrastructure of human atheroma. Exp. molec. Path. *7:* 378–400 (1967).
89 GILLMAN, J. and GILBERT, C.: Atherosis in the baboon *(Papio ursinus)*. Its pathogenesis and etiology. Exp. Med. Surg. *15:* 181–221 (1957).
90 GILLOT, P.: Les altérations histologiques des coronaires fœtales et infantiles. Acta cardiol. *17:* 145–165 (1962).
91 GLAGOV, S.: Hemodynamic factors in localization of atherosclerosis. Acta cardiol. (suppl.) *11:* 311–337 (1965).
92 GORDON, I.: Mechanism of lipophage deposition in atherosclerosis. Arch. Path. *44:* 247–260 (1947).
93 GREENLEE, T. K., jr.; ROOS, R., and HARTMAN, J. L.: The fine structure of elastic fibers. J. Cell Biol. *30:* 59–71 (1966).
94 GREIG, H. B. W.: Inhibition of fibrinolysis by alimentary lipemia. Lancet *ii:* 16–18 (1956).
95 GROSS, L.; EPSTEIN, E. Z., and KUGEL, M. A.: Histology of the coronary arteries and their branches in the human heart. Amer. J. Path. *10:* 253–274 (1934).
96 GROSS, R. E. and WOLBACH, S. B.: Sclerosing hemangiomas. Amer. J. Path. *19:* 533–544 (1943).
97 GRÜNSTEIN, N.: Über den Bau der grösseren menschlichen Arterien in verschiedenen Altersstufen. Arch. mikroskop. Anat. *47:* 583–654 (1896).
98 HAND, R. A. and CHANDLER, A. B.: Atherosclerotic metamorphosis of autologous pulmonary thrombo-emboli in the rabbit. Amer. J. Path. *40:* 469–486 (1962).
99 HARRIS, P. N.: Are foamy cells in atheromata of reticuloendothelial origin? Proc. Soc. exp. Biol., N.Y. *79:* 455–456 (1952).
100 HARRISON, C. V.: Experimental pulmonary arteriosclerosis. J. Path. Bact. *60:* 289–293 (1948).

101 HARTROFT, W. S.; RIDOUT, J. H.; SELLERS, E. A., and BEST, C. M.: Atheromatous changes in aorta, carotid and coronary arteries of choline-deficient rats. Proc. Soc. exp. Biol., N.Y. *81:* 384–393 (1952).

102 HASS, G. M.; TRUEHEART, R. E., and HEMMENS, A.: Experimental athero-arteriosclerosis due to calcific medial degeneration and hypercholesteremia. Amer. J. Path. *38:* 289–329 (1961).

103 HASSLER, O.: The origin of the cells constituting arterial intima thickening. An experimental autoradiographic study with the use of H^3-Thymidine. Lab. Invest. *22:* 286–293 (1970).

104 HAUST, M. D.; MOVAT, H. Z., and MORE, R. H.: The role of fibrin thrombi in the genesis of the common white plaque in ateriosclerosis. Circulation *14:* 483 (1956).

105 HAUST, M. D. and MORE, R. H.: Morphologic evidence and significance of permeation in the genesis of arteriosclerosis. Circulation *16:* 496 (1957).

106 HAUST, M. D.; MOVAT, H. Z., and MORE, R. H.: Organization by smooth muscle cells. Amer. J. Path. *33:* 626 (1957).

107 HAUST, M. D. and MORE, R. H.: New functional aspects of smooth muscle cells. Fed. Proc. *17:* 440 (1958).

108 HAUST, M. D.; MORE, R. H., and MOVAT, H. Z.: The mechanism of fibrosis in arteriosclerosis. Amer. J. Path. *35:* 265–273 (1959).

109 HAUST, M. D.; MORE, R. H., and MOVAT, H. Z.: The role of smooth muscle cells in the fibrogenesis of arteriosclerosis. Amer. J. Path. *37:* 377–389 (1960).

110 HAUST, M. D. and MORE, R. H.: The thrombotic basis of arteriosclerosis. Heart Bull. *9:* 90–92 (1960).

111 HAUST, M. D.; BALIS, J. U., and MORE, R. H.: Electron microscopic study of intimal lipid accumulations in human aorta and their pathogenesis. Circulation *26:* 656 (1962).

112 HAUST, M. D. and MORE, R. H.: Significance of the smooth muscle cell in atherogenesis; in JONES Evolution of the atherosclerotic plaque, pp. 51–63 (University of Chicago Press, Chicago 1963).

113 HAUST, M. D.; MORE, R. H.; BENCOSME, S. A., and BALIS, J. U.: Elastogenesis in human aorta: an electron microscopic study. Exp. molec. Path. *4:* 508–524 (1965).

114 HAUST, M. D.; WYLLIE, J. C., and MORE, R. H.: Electron microscopy of fibrin in human atherosclerotic lesions. Immunohistochemical and morphologic identification. Exp. molec. Path. *4:* 205–216 (1965).

115 HAUST, M. D.: Fine fibrils of extracellular space (microfibrils). Amer. J. Path. *47:* 1113–1137 (1965).

116 HAUST, M. D. and MORE, R. H.: Mechanism of fibrosis in white atherosclerotic plaque of human aorta. An electron microscopic study. Circulation *34:* 14 (1966).

117 HAUST, M. D.; MORE, R. H.; BENCOSME, S. A., and BALIS, J. U.: Electron microscopic studies in human atherosclerosis. Extracellular elements in aortic dots and streaks. Exp. molec. Path. *6:* 300–313 (1967).

118 HAUST, M. D. and MORE, R. H.: Electron microscopy of connective tissues and elastogenesis. International Academy of Pathology, monogr. No. 7, The connective tissues, pp. 352–376 (Williams and Wilkins, Baltimore 1967).

119 HAUST, M. D.: Injury and repair in the pathogenesis of atherosclerosis; in JONES Atherosclerosis. Proc. 2nd Int. Symp., pp. 12–20 (Springer, New York 1970).

120 Haust, M. D.: The morphogenesis and fate of potential and early atherosclerotic lesions in man. Human Path. *2:* 1–29 (1971).

121 Haust, M. D.: Arteriosclerosis; in Brunson and Gall Concepts of disease. A textbook of human pathology, pp. 451–487 (Macmillan, New York 1971).

122 Haust, M. D.: Platelet-fibrin microthrombi of aortic intima of normal rabbits. Unpublished observations (1971).

123 Heard, B. E.: An experimental study of thickening of the pulmonary arteries of rabbits produced by the organization of fibrin. J. Path. Bact. *64:* 13–19 (1952).

124 Heath, D.; DuShane, J. W.; Wood, E. H., and Edwards, J. E.: The structure of the pulmonary trunk at different ages and in cases of pulmonary hypertension and pulmonary stenosis. J. Path. Bact. *77:* 443–456 (1959).

125 Hepinstall, R. H.: The effects of high blood cholesterol on the pulmonary arterial changes produced in rabbits by the injection of blood clot. Brit. J. exp. Path. *38:* 438–445 (1957).

126 Hieronymi, G.: Über den altersbedingten Formwandel elastischer und muskulärer Arterien. Österr. Akad. Wiss., math.-naturw. SitzBer., pp. 221–352 (1956).

127 Hirsch, S.: L'athérome aortique des enfants: études à propos des débuts de la soidisant artériosclérose. Cardiologia *5:* 122–188 (1942).

128 Hoff, H. F.: A comparison on the fine-structural localization of nucleoside phosphatase activity in large intracranial blood vessels and the thoracic aorta of rabbits. Histochemie *13:* 183–191 (1968).

129 Hoff, H. F.; McDonald, L. W., and Hayes, T. L.: An electron microscope study of the rabbit aortic intima after occlusion by brief exposure to a single ligature. Brit. J. exp. Path. *49:* 68–73 (1968).

130 Hoff, H. F. and Gottlob, R.: Ultrastructural changes of large rabbit blood vessels following mild mechanical trauma. Virchows Arch. path. Anat. *345:* 93–106 (1968).

131 Hueper, W. C.: Experimental studies in cardiovascular pathology. Pectin atheromatosis and thesaurosis in rabbits and in dogs. Arch. Path. *34:* 883–901 (1942).

132 Hueper, W. C.: Arteriosclerosis. A general review. Arch. Path. *38:* 162–181, 245–285, 326–328, 350–364, 381–391 (1944).

133 Hüttner, I.; More, R. H., and Rona, G.: Fine structural evidence of specific mechanism for increased endothelial permeability in experimental hypertension. Amer. J. Path. *61:* 395–412 (1970).

134 Imai, H.; Lee, K. J.; Lee, S. K.; Lee, K. T.; O'Neal, R. M., and Thomas, W. A.: Ultrastructural features of aortic cells in mitosis in control and cholesterol-fed swine. Lab. Invest. *23:* 401–415 (1970).

135 Jennings, M. A.; Florey, H. W.; Stehbens, W. E., and French, J. E.: Intimal changes in the arteries of a pig. J. Path. Bact. *81:* 49–61 (1961).

136 Jensen, J. G.: An electron microscopic study on the morphology of the elastin in foetal, human aortas. Acta path. microbiol. scand. *56:* 388–398 (1962).

137 Jones, R. J.: Evolution of the atherosclerotic plaque (University of Chicago Press, Chicago 1963).

138 Jores, L.: Zur Frage des postembryonalen Gefässwachstums. Dtsch. med. Wschr. *48:* 649–650 (1922).

139 Jores, L.: Arterien; in Henke and Lubarsch Handbuch der speziellen pathologischen Anatomie und Histologie, vol. 2: Herz und Gefässe, pp. 608–786 (Springer, Berlin 1924).

140 Jorgensen, L.; Rowsell, H. C.; Hovig, T., and Mustard, J. F.: Resolution and organization of platelet-rich mural thrombi in carotid arteries of swine. Amer. J. Path. *51:* 681–719 (1967).
141 Jurukova, Z.: Elektronenmikroskopische Untersuchungen über die Beteiligung glatter Muskelzellen der Arterienwand an der Organisation arterieller Thromben. Verh. dtsch. ges. Path. *53:* 464–469 (1969).
142 Jurukova, Z. und Knieriem, H. J.: Elektronenmikroskopische Untersuchungen über die Organisation arterieller Thromben. Virchows Arch. path. Anat. *349:* 368–381 (1970).
143 Kádár, A.; Veress, B., and Jellinek, H.: Ultrastructural elements in experimental intimal thickening. II. Study of the development of elastic elements in intimal proliferation. Exp. molec. Path. *11:* 212–223 (1969).
144 Kaplan, D. and Meyer, K.: Mucopolysaccharides of aorta at various ages. Proc. Soc. exp. Biol. N.Y. *105:* 78–81 (1960).
145 Karrer, H. E.: Electron microscope study of developing chick embryo aorta. J. Ultrastruct. Res. *4:* 420–454 (1960).
146 Karrer, H. E.: An electron microscopic study of the aorta in young and in aging mice. J. Ultrastruct. Res. *5:* 1–27 (1961).
147 Keech, M. K.: Electron microscope study of the lathyritic rat aorta. J. biophys. biochem. Cytol. *7:* 539–546 (1959).
148 Keech, M. K.: Electron microscope study of the normal rat aorta. J. biophys. biochem. Cytol. *7:* 533–538 (1960).
149 Klotz, O.: Concerning compensatory hyperplasia of the intima. J. exp. Med. *12:* 707–725 (1910).
150 Klotz, O.: Nodular endarteritis of the aorta about the intercostal arteries. J. med. Res. *31:* 409–429 (1914–1915).
151 Klotz, O.: Fatty degeneration of the intima of arteries. J. med. Res. *32:* 27–43 (1915).
152 Knieriem, H. J.; Kao, V. C. Y., and Wissler, R. W.: Actomyosin and myosin and the deposition of lipids and serum lipoproteins. Arch. Path. *84:* 118–129 (1967).
153 Kölliker, A.: Handbuch der Gewebelehre des Menschen; 5th ed. (Engelmann, Leipzig 1867).
154 Krause, C.: Zur Frage der Arteriosklerose bei Rind, Pferd und Hund. Beitr. path. Anat. *70:* 121–178 (1922).
155 Kuntz, A. and Sulkin, N. M.: Lesions induced in rabbits by cholesterol feeding, with special reference to their origin. Arch. Path. *47:* 248–260 (1949).
156 Laguens, R. and Lagrutta, J.: Fine structure of human uterine muscle in pregnancy. Amer. J. Obstet. Gynec. *89:* 1040–1048 (1964).
157 Laing, W.; Rowsell, H., and Mustard, F.: Morphological studies of pig's aorta. Abstract. Anat. Rec. *145:* 251 (1963).
158 Laitinen, E.: Changes in the elemental structures of the aorta in human and experimental atherosclerosis. Light and electron microscopic studies. Acta path. microbiol. scand. (suppl.) *161–167:* 1–92 (1963).
159 Langhans, Th.: Beiträge zur normalen und pathologischen Anatomie der Arterien. Virchows Arch. path. Anat. *36:* 187–226 (1866).
160 Leary, T.: Atherosclerosis. Special consideration of aortic lesions. Arch. Path. *21:* 419–458 (1936).
161 Leary, T.: The genesis of atherosclerosis. Arch. Path. *32:* 507–555 (1941).

162 Lee, K. T.; Lee, K. J.; Lee, S. K.; Imai, H., and O Neal, R. M.: Poorly differentiated subendothelial cells in swine aortas. Exp. molec. Path. *13:* 118–129 (1970).

163 Lev, M. and Sullivan, C. M.: The relationship of ageing changes to the development of arteriosclerosis in human aorta. Abstract. Amer. J. Path. *27:* 648–686 (1951).

164 Levene, C. I.: The early lesions of atheroma in the coronary arteries. J. Path. Bact. *72:* 79–82 (1956).

165 Lewis, W. H. and Lewis, M. R.: Behavior of cells in tissue cultures; in Cowdry General cytology (University of Chicago Press, Chicago 1924).

166 Lindsay, S.; Chaikoff, I. L. and Gilmore, J. W.: Arteriosclerosis in the dog. I. Spontaneous lesions in the aorta and the coronary arteries. Arch. Path. *53:* 281–300 (1952).

167 Lindsay, S. and Chaikoff, I. L.: Arteriosclerosis in the baboon. Naturally occurring lesions in the aorta and coronary and iliac arteries. Arch. Path. *63:* 460–471 (1957).

168 Lober, P. H.: Pathogenesis of coronary sclerosis. Arch. Path. *55:* 357–383 (1953).

169 Majno, G.; Shea, S. M., and Leventhal, M.: Endothelial contraction induced by histamine-type mediators: an electron microscopic study. J. Cell Biol. *42:* 647–672 (1969).

170 Mallory, F. B.: The infectious lesions of blood vessels. The Harvey Lectures, 1912–1913 p. 150 (Lippincott Philadelphia 1913).

171 Malyschew B. F.: Über die Reaktion des Endothels der Art. carotis des Kaninchens bei doppelter Unterbindung. Virchows Arch. path. Anat. *272:* 727–752 (1929).

172 Mandel, E. E.; Rosenthal W. and Roth H.: Lipemia-induced acceleration of intra-vascular clotting. Clin. Res. *6:* 394–395 (1958).

173 Manley, G.: Changes in vascular mucopolysaccharides with age and blood pressure. Brit. J. exp. Path. *46:* 125–134 (1965).

174 Marchand, F.: in Eulenburg Realenzyklopädie der gesamten Heilkunde vol. 1, p. 768 (Urban & Schwarzenberg, Berlin 1907).

175 Marshall, J. R. and O'Neal, R. M.: The lipophage in hyperlipemic rats: an electron microscopic study. Exp. molec. Path. *5:* 1–11 (1966).

176 Marshall, J. R.; Adams, J. G.; O'Neal, R. M., and DeBakey, M. E.: The ultrastructure of uncomplicated human atheroma in surgically resected aortas. J. Atheroscler. Res. *6:* 120–131 (1966).

177 Maruffo, C. A. and Portman, O. W.: Nutritional control of coronary artery atherosclerosis in the squirrel monkey. J. Atheroscler. Res. *8:* 237–247 (1968).

178 Masloff, M. S.: Zur Frage über die Entwicklung der grossen Gefässe (der Aorta und der Art. brachialis) beim menschlichen Embryo. Arch. mikroskop. Anat. *84:* 351–368 (1914).

179 Maximow, A.: Behavior of endothelium of blood vessels in tissue culture. Anat. Rec. *29:* 369 (1925).

180 McCombs, H. L.; Zook, B. C., and McGandy, R. B.: Fine structure of spontaneous atherosclerosis of the aorta in squirrel monkey. Amer. J. Path. *55:* 235–252 (1969).

181 McLetchie, N. G. B.: The pathogenesis of atheroma. Amer. J. Path. *28:* 413–435 (1952).

182 McMillan, G. C. and Duff, G. L.: Mitotic activity in the aortic lesions of experimental cholesterol atherosclerosis of rabbits. Arch. Path. *46:* 179–182 (1948).

183 McMillan, G. C.: The onset of plaque formation in arteriosclerosis. Acta cardiol. (suppl.) *11:* 43–62 (1965).

184 McMILLAN, G. C. and STARY, H. C.: Preliminary experience with mitotic activity of cellular elements in the atherosclerotic plaques of cholesterol-fed rabbits studied by labeling with tritiated thymidine. Ann. N.Y. Acad. Sci. *149:* 699–712 (1968).

185 MEYER, W. W.: Die Bedeutung der Eiweissablagerungen in der Histogenese arteriosklerotischer Intima-Veränderungen der Aorta. Virchows Arch. path. Anat. *316:* 268–316 (1949).

186 MEYER, W. W.: Die Lebenswandlung der Struktur von Arterien und Venen. Verh. dtsch. Ges. KreislForsch. *24:* 15–40 (1958).

187 MINKOWSKI, W.: The coronary arteries of infants. Amer. J. med. Sci. *214:* 623–629 (1947).

188 MOON, H. D. and RINEHART, J. F.: Histogenesis of coronary arteriosclerosis. Circulation *6:* 481–488 (1952),

189 MOON, H. D.: Coronary arteries in fetuses, infants, and juveniles. Circulation *16:* 263–267 (1957).

190 MORE, R. H. and HAUST, M. D.: Encrustation and permeation of blood proteins in the genesis of arteriosclerosis. Amer. J. Path. *33:* 593 (1957)

191 MORE, R. H.; MOVAT, H. Z., and HAUST, M. D.: Role of mural fibrin thrombi of the aorta in genesis of arteriosclerotic plaques. Arch. Path. *63:* 612–620 (1957).

192 MORE, R. H. and HAUST. M. D.: Atherogenesis and plasma constituents. Amer. J. Path. *38:* 527–537 (1961).

193 MORE, R. H. and HAUST. M. D.: Diffuse intimal thickening of coronary arteries in children and young adults and its role in atherosclerosis; in Le rôle de la paroi artérielle dans l'athérogénèse. Coll. Int., C.N.R.S., Paris No. 169. pp. 75–91 (1968).

194 MOREHEAD. R. P. and LITTLE. J. M.: Changes in the blood vessels of apparently healthy mongrel dogs. Amer. J. Path. *21:* 339–355 (1945)

195 MORELAND, A. F.: Atherosclerosis in 'miniture' swine. Arch. Path *76:* 203–211 (1963)

196 MORGAN, A. D.: The pathogenesis of coronary occlusion (Blackwell, Oxford 1956)

197 MOSS, N. S. and BENDITT, E. P.: Spontaneous and experimentally induced arterial lesions. I. An ultrastructural survey of the normal chicken aorta. Lab. Invest. *22:* 166–183 (1970).

198 MOSS, N. S. and BENDITT, E. P.: The ultrastructure of spontaneous and experimentally induced arterial lesions. III. The cholesterol-induced lesions and the effect of a cholesterol and oil diet on the preexisting spontaneous plaque in the chicken aorta. Lab. Invest. *23:* 231–245 (1970).

199 MOSS, N. S. and BENDITT, E. P.: The ultrastructure of spontaneous and experimentally induced arterial lesions. II. The spontaneous plaque in the chicken. Lab. Invest. *23:* 521–535 (1970).

200 MOVAT, H. Z.; MORE, R. H., and HAUST, M. D.: The diffuse intimal thickening of the human aorta with ageing. Amer. J. Path. *34:* 1023–1031 (1958).

201 MOVAT, H. Z.; HAUST, M. D., and MORE, R. H.: The morphologic elements in the early lesions of arteriosclerosis. Amer. J. Path. *35:* 93–101 (1959).

202 MÜLLER, E. and FRIEDLEIN, M.: Messergebnisse bei coronarsklerotischem Mediaschwund und Intimaumbau und ihre Bedeutung für die vasomotorische Durchblutungsregelung. Frankf. Z. Path. *69:* 268–278 (1958).

203 MURPHY, E. A.; ROWSELL, H. C.; DOWNIE, H. G.; ROBINSON, G. A., and MUSTARD J. F.: Encrustation and atherosclerosis: the analogy between early *in vivo* lesions and deposits which occur in extracorporeal circulations. Canad. med. Ass. J. *87:* 259–274 (1962).

204 MURRAY, M.; SCHRODT, G. R., and BERG, H. F.: Role of smooth muscle in cells in healing of injured arteries. Arch. Path. *82:* 138–146 (1966).

205 MUSTARD, J. F.: Recent advances in molecular pathology: a review. Platelet aggregation, vascular injury and atherosclerosis. Exp. molec. Path. *7:* 366–377 (1967).

206 NACHMAN, R.; MARCUS, A. J., and SAFIER, L. B.: Platelet thrombosthenin: subcellular localization and function. J. clin. Invest. *46:* 1380–1389 (1967).

207 NEUFELD, H. N.; WAGENVOORT, C. A., and EDWARDS, J. E.: Coronary arteries in fetuses, infants, juveniles, and young adults. Lab. Invest. *11:* 837–844 (1962).

208 NEWMAN, H. A. I. and ZILVERSMIT, D. B.: Quantitative aspects of cholesterol flux in rabbit atheromatous lesions. J. biol. Chem. *237:* 2078–2984 (1962).

209 O'NEAL, R. M.; STILL, W. J. S., and HARTROFT, W. S.: Experimental atherosclerosis in the rat. J. Path. Bact. *82:* 183–188 (1961).

210 O'NEAL, R. M.; JORDAN, G. L., jr.; DE BAKEY, M. E., and HALPERT, B.: Cells grown on isolated intravascular dacron hub. An electron microscopic study. Exp. molec. Path. *3:* 403–412 (1964).

211 OPPENHEIM, F.: Über den histologischen Bau der Arterien in der wachsenden und alternden Niere. Frankf. Z. Path. *21:* 57–84 (1918).

212 PALLASKE, G.: Atherosklerose beim Papagei. Frankf. Z. Path. *40:* 64–80 (1930).

213 PARKER, F.: An electron microscope study of coronary arteries. Amer. J. Anat. *103:* 247–273 (1958).

214 PARKER, F.: An electron microscopic study of experimental atherosclerosis. Amer. J. Path. *36:* 19–53 (1960).

215 PARKER, F. and ODLAND, G. F.: A correlative histochemical, biochemical, and electron microscopic study of experimental atherosclerosis in the rabbit aorta with special reference to the myo-intimal cell. Amer. J. Path. *48:* 197–239 (1966).

216 PATERSON, J. C.; MILLS, J., and LOCKWOOD, C. H.: The role of hypertension in progression of atherosclerosis. Canad. med. Ass. J. *82:* 65–70 (1960).

217 PAULE, W. J.: Electron microscopy of the newborn rat aorta. J. Ultrastruct. Res. *8:* 219–235 (1963).

218 PEASE, D. C. and PAULE, W. J.: Electron microscopy of elastic arteries; the thoracic aorta of the rat. J. Ultrastruct. Res. *3:* 469–483 (1960).

219 PEASE, D. C. and MOLINARI, S.: Electron microscopy of muscular arteries; pial vessels of the cat and monkey. J. Ultrastruct. Res. *3:* 447–468 (1960).

220 PICKERING, G. W.: Arteriosclerosis and atherosclerosis. The need for clear thinking. Amer. J. Med. *34:* 7–18 (1963).

221 PICKERING, G. W.: Pathogenesis of myocardial and cerebral infarction: nodular arteriosclerosis. Brit. med. J. *i:* 517–528 (1964).

222 POLZER, C.; STUDER A. and HESS R.: Symposium on Duguid's hypothesis. Bull. Swiss Acad. med. Sci. *22* (4)*:* 1–12 (1966).

223 POOLE J. C. F. and ROBINSON D. S.: Further observations on the effects of ethanolamine phosphatide on plasma coagulation. Quart. J. exp. Physiol. *41:* 295–300 (1956).

224 POOLE J. C. F. and FLOREY H. W.: Changes in the endothelium of the aorta and the behavior of macrophages in experimental atheroma of rabbits. J. Path. Bact. *75:* 245–251 (1958).
225 POOLE J. C. F.; CROMWELL S. B. and BENDITT E. P.: Behavior of smooth muscle cells and formation of extracellular structures in the reaction of arterial walls to injury. Amer. J. Path. *62:* 391–413 (1971).
226 PRIOR J. T. and JONES D. B.: Structural alterations within the aortic intima in infancy and childhood. Amer. J. Path. *28:* 937–951 (1952).
227 PUCHTLER H.; SWEAT F.; TERRY M. S. and CONNER H. M.: Investigation of staining polarization and fluorescence-microscopic properties of myoendothelial cells. J. Microscopy *89:* 95–104 (1968).
228 RANNIE I. and DUGUID J. B.: The pathogenesis of cholesterol arteriosclerosis in the rabbit. J. Path. Bact. *66:* 395–398 (1953).
229 RHODIN J. A. G.: Fine structure of vascular walls in mammals with special reference to smooth muscle component. Physiol. Rev. *42:* suppl. vol. 5, pp. 48–87 (1962).
230 RIBBERT, H.: Über die Genese der arteriosklerotischen Veränderungen der Intima Verh. dtsch. Ges. Path. *8:* 168–177 (1904).
231 ROBERT, L.: The macromolecular matrix of the arterial wall: collagen, elastin, mucopolysaccharides; in JONES Atherosclerosis. Proc. 2nd Int. Symp., pp. 59–68 (Springer, New York 1970).
232 ROBERTSON, J. H.: Stress zones in foetal arteries. J. clin. Path. *13:* 133–139 (1960).
233 ROBERTSON, J. H.: The influence of mechanical factors on the structure of the peripheral arteries and the localization of atherosclerosis. J. clin. Path. *13:* 199–204 (1960).
234 ROBERTSON, J. H.: The significance of intimal thickening in the arteries of the newborn. Arch. Dis. Childh. *35:* 588–590 (1960).
235 ROBERTSON, W. B.; GEER, J. C.; STRONG, J. P., and MCGILL, H. C., jr.: The fate of the fatty streak. Exp. molec. Path. (suppl.) *1:* 28–39 (1963).
236 ROKITANSKY, C. VON: A manual of pathological anatomy, vol. 4 (Sydenham, London 1852).
237 ROSEN, L.; BOWDEN, D. H., and UCHIDA, I.: Structural changes in pulmonary arteries in first year of life. Arch. Path. *63:* 316–317 (1957).
238 ROSS, R. and BORNSTEIN, P.: The elastic fiber. I. Separation and partial characterization of its macromolecular components. J. Cell Biol. *40:* 366–381 (1969).
239 ROSS, R.; EVERETT, N. B., and TYLER, R.: Wound healing and collagen formation. VI. The origin of the wound fibroblast studied in parabiosis. J. Cell Biol. *44:* 645–654 (1970).
240 ROSSLE, R.: Über die serösen Entzündungen der Organe. Virchows Arch. path. Anat. *311:* 252–284 (1944).
241 SAKO, Y. and NAKAMURA, M.: Electron microscopic studies on the rabbit aorta in acute hypercholesterolemia. Jap. Heart J. *4:* 53–68 (1963).
242 SALDANA, M. and ARIAS-STELLA, J.: Studies on the structure of the pulmonary trunk. I. Normal changes in the elastic configuration of the human pulmonary trunk and different ages. Circulation *27:* 1086–1093 (1963).
243 SALGADO, E. D.: Medial aortic lesions in rats with metacorticoid hypertension. Amer. J. Path. *58:* 305–327 (1970).
244 SAPPINGTON, S. W. and COOK, H. S.: Radial artery changes in comparison with those of the coronary and other arteries. Amer. J. med. Sci. *192:* 822–839 (1936).

245 SAPPINGTON, S. W. and HORNEFF, J. A.: Tibial artery changes in comparison with those of the radial and coronary arteries. Amer. J. med. Sci. *201:* 862–871 (1941).

246 SCHÖNHEIMER, R.: Experimentelle Venen-Atherosklerose. Virchows Arch. path. Anat. *251:* 732–738 (1924).

247 SCHORNAGEL, H. E.: Intimal thickening in the coronary arteries in infants. Arch. Path. *62:* 427–432 (1956).

248 SCOTT, R. F.; FLORENTIN, R. A.; DAOUD, A. S.; MORRISON, E. S.; JONES, R. M., and HUTT, M. S. R.: Coronary arteries of children and young adults. A comparison of lipids and anatomic features in New Yorkers and East Africans. Exp. molec. Path. *5:* 12–42 (1966).

249 SENDRAIL-PESQUE, M.; JULIAN, M.; DURROUX, R.; FABRE, M. T.; RUMEAU, J. L. et BOUISSOU, H.: Le vieillissement aortique. Path. Biol. *17:* 223–234 (1969).

250 SHEEHAN, J. F.: Foam cell plaques in the intima of irradiated small arteries (one hundred to five hundred microns in external diameter). Arch. Path. *37:* 297–308 (1944).

251 SHIMAMOTO, T.: The relationship of edematous reaction in arteries to atherosclerosis and thrombosis. J. Atheroscler. Res. *3:* 87–102 (1963).

252 SHIMAMOTO, T.; MAEZAWA, H.; YAMAZAKI, H.; ISHIOKA, T.; SUNAGA, T., and FUJITA, T.: Edematous arterial reaction and its relationship to atherosclerosis and thrombosis. Meth. Achievem. exp. Path., vol. 1, p. 337 (Karger, Basel 1966).

253 SHIMAMOTO, T.: Experimental study on atherosclerosis – an attempt at its prevention and treatment. Acta path. jap. *19:* 15–43 (1969).

254 SHIMAMURA, T.: Ultrastructural studies of the medial aortic sclerosis in rats with experimentally induced chronic renal disease. Exp. molec. Path. *13:* 79–88 (1970).

255 SHORE, M. L.; ZILVERSMIT, D. B., and ACKERMAN, R. F.: Plasma phospholipide deposition and aortic phospholipide synthesis in experimental atherosclerosis. Amer. J. Physiol. *181:* 527–531 (1955).

256 SILBERBERG, M.: Endothel in der Gewebskultur. Arch. exp. Zellforsch. *9:* 36–53 (1929).

257 SIMON, R. C.; STILL, W. J. S., and O'NEAL, R. M.: The circulating lipophage and experimental atherosclerosis. J. Atheroscler. Res. *1:* 395–400 (1961).

258 SIMONTON, J. H. and GOFMAN, J. M.: Microphage migration in experimental atherosclerosis. Circulation *4:* 557–562 (1951).

259 SIMPSON, C. F. and HARMS, R. H.: The nature of the atherosclerotic plaque in the turkey. J. Atheroscler. Res. *8:* 143–153 (1968).

260 SIMPSON, C. F. and HARMS, R. H.: Aortic atherosclerosis of turkeys induced by feeding of cholesterol. J. Atheroscler. Res. *10:* 63–75 (1969).

261 SPALTEHOLZ, W. und HOCHREIN, M.: Untersuchungen am Koronarsystem der anatomischen und funktionellen Beschaffenheit der Koronararterienwand. Arch. exp. Path. Pharmakol. *163:* 333–352 (1931–1932).

262 SPARAGEN, S. C.; BOND, V. P. and DAHL, L. K.: The role of hyperplasia in vascular lesions of cholesterol-fed rabbits studied with thymidine-H^3 autoradiography. Circulat. Res. *11:* 329–336 (1962).

263 STEHBENS, W. E.: Focal intimal proliferation in the cerebral arteries. Amer. J. Path. *36:* 289–301 (1960).

264 STILL, W. J. S. and O'NEIL, R. M.: Electron microscopic study of experimental atherosclerosis in the rat. Amer. J. Path. *40:* 21–35 (1962).

265 STILL, W. J. S. and MARRIOTT, P. R.: Comparative morphology of the early atherosclerotic lesion in man and cholesterol-atherosclerosis in the rabbit. An electron microscope study. J. Atheroscler. Res. *4:* 373–386 (1964).

266 STILL, W. J. S.: An electron microscopic study of the organization of experimental thromboemboli in the rabbit. Lab. Invest. *15:* 1492–1507 (1966).

267 STILL, W. J. S.; GHANI, A. R., and DENNISON, S. M.: The organization of isolated mural thrombi in aortic grafts. An electron microscopic study. Amer. J. Path. *51:* 1013–1029 (1967).

268 STRONG, K. C. A.: A study of the structure of the media of the distributing arteries by the method of microdissection. Anat. Rec. *72:* 151–167 (1938).

269 STUDER, A. und LOREZ, H. P.: Intravasale Fibrinbildung und ihre Beziehung zur normalen und veränderten Aorta des Kaninchens. Path. Microbiol. *28:* 738–750 (1965).

270 STUMPF, R.: Über die Entartungsvorgänge in der Aorta des Kindes und ihre Beziehungen zur Atherosklerose. Beitr. path. Anat. *59:* 390–417 (1914).

271 SUZUKI, M. and O'NEAL, R. M.: Accumulation of lipids in the leukocytes of rats fed atherogenic diets. J. Lipid Res. *5:* 624–627 (1964).

272 TAYLOR, C. B.; BALDWIN, D., and HASS, G. M.: Localized arteriosclerotic lesions induced in the aorta of the juvenile rabbit by freezing. Arch. Path. *49:* 623–640 (1950).

273 THOMAS, W. A.; JONES, R.; SCOTT, R. F.; MORRISON, E.; GOODALE, F., and IMAI, H.: Production of early atherosclerotic lesions in rats characterized by proliferation of 'modified smooth muscle cells'. Exp. molec. Path. (suppl.) 1–2*:* 40–61 (1963).

274 TORHORST, H.: Die histologischen Veränderungen bei der Sklerose der Pulmonalarterie. Beitr. path. Anat. *36:* 210–241 (1904).

275 TRAUTMANN, A. and FIEBIGER, J.: Fundamentals of the histology of domestic animals (translated and revised from the 8th and 9th German edition, by HABEL and BIBERSTEIN) (Baillière, Tindall & Cox, London 1952/Comstock Publishing Associates, Ithaca 1952).

276 TRILLO, A.; RENAUD, S., and HAUST, M. D.: Ultrastructure of aortic lesions in normotensive and hypertensive hyperlipemic rats. Fed. Proc. *29:* 487 (1970).

277 TS'AO, C. and GLAGOV, S.: Basal endothelial attachment. Tenacity at cytoplasmic dense zones in rabbit aorta. Lab. Invest. *23:* 510–516 (1970).

278 UOTILA, U.; LEVONEN, E., and RAEKALLIO, J.: On the effect of atherosclerosis and goitre on aortic histopathology and mucopolysaccharide content. Acta endocrin., Kbh. *36:* 1-8 (1961).

279 USUKU, G.; SIMONAGAYOSI, S.; KODAMA, Y. and ARATAKE, H.: Ultrastructure of the lamina elastica interna of rabbit's femoral artery. Kumamoto med. J. *12:* 285–287 (1959).

280 VERESS, B.; KÁDÁR, A., and JELLINEK, H.: Ultrastructural elements in experimental intimal thickening. I. Electron microscopic study of the development and cellular elements of intimal proliferation. Exp. molec. Path. *11:* 200–211 (1969).

281 VERSÉ, M.: Zur Frage der experimentellen Atherosklerose. Zbl. allg. Path. path. Anat. *34:* 614–615 (1924).

282 VIRCHOW, R.: Phlogose und Thrombose im Gefäss-System. Gesammelte Abhandlungen zur wissenschaftlichen Medicin (Meidinger, Frankfurt 1856).

283 VIRCHOW, R.: Die Cellularpathologie. 4th ed. (Hirschwald, Berlin 1871).

284 Vlodaver, Z. and Neufeld, H. N.: The musculo-elastic layer in the coronary arteries. A histological and hemodynamic concept. Vasc. Dis. *4–5:* 136–145 (1967–1968).
285 Vlodaver, Z.; Kahn, H. A., and Neufeld, H. N.: The coronary arteries in early life in three different ethnic groups. Circulation *39:* 541–550 (1969).
286 Wacker, L. and Hueck, W.: Über experimentelle Atherosklerose und Cholesterinaemie. Münch. med. Wschr. *60:* 2097–2100 (1913).
287 Wagenvoort, C. A. and Wagenvoort, N.: Age changes in muscular pulmonary arteries. Arch. Path. *79:* 524–528 (1965).
288 Watts, H.: Basic aspects of the pathogenesis of human atherosclerosis. Human Path. *2:* 31–55 (1971).
289 Weibel, E. R. and Palade, G. E.: New cytoplasmic components in arterial endothelia. J. Cell Biol. *23:* 101–112 (1964).
290 Westlake, G. E.; Grundy, S. M., and O'Neal, R. M.: The effect of an atherogeneic diet on pre-existing aortic intimal thickenings in old dogs. Exp. molec. Path. (suppl.) *1:* 1–8 (1963).
291 Wilens, S. L.: The nature of diffuse intimal thickening of arteries. Amer. J. Path. *27:* 825–839 (1951).
292 Willius, F. A.; Smith, H. L., and Sprague, P. H.: A study of coronary and aortic sclerosis: incidence and degree in 5,060 consecutive postmortem examinations. Proc. Staff Meet. Mayo Clin. *8:* 140–144 (1933).
293 Wissler, R. W.; Frazier, L. E.; Hughes, R. H., and Rasmussen, R. H.: Atherogenesis in the Cebus monkey. I. A comparison of three food fats under controlled dietary conditions. Arch. Path. *74:* 312–322 (1962).
294 Woerner, C. A.: Endothelial reaction to intravenous lipids. Anat. Rec. *109:* 360 (1951).
295 Wolinsky, H. and Glagov, S.: Comparison of abdominal and thoracic aortic medial structure in mammals. Deviation of man from the usual pattern. Circulat. Res. *25:* 677–686 (1969).
296 Wolinsky, H. and Glagov, S.: Nature of species differences in the medial distribution of aortic vasa vasorum in mammals. Circulat. Res. *20:* 409–421 (1967).
297 Wolinsky, H.: Comparison of medial growth of human thoracic and abdominal aortas. Circulat. Res. *27:* 531–538 (1970).
298 Wolkoff, K.: Über die histologische Structur der Coronararterien des menschlichen Herzens. Virchows Arch. path. Anat. *241–243:* 42–58 (1923).
299 Wolkoff, K.: Über die Altersveränderungen der Arterien bei Tieren. Virchows Arch. path. Anat. *252:* 208–228 (1924).
300 Wolkoff, K.: Über die Atherosklerose der Coronararterien des Herzens. Zieglers Beiträge: vide Beitr. path. Anat. *82:* 555–596 (1929).
301 Wright, I.: The microscopical appearances of human peripheral arteries during growth and aging. J. clin. Path. *16:* 499–522 (1963).
302 Zinserling, W. D.: Über die pathologischen Veränderungen der Aorta beim Pferde in Verbindung mit der Lehre der Atherosklerose beim Menschen. Virchows Arch. path. Anat. *213:* 23–41 (1913).
303 Zinserling, W. D.: Vergleichend-morphologische Untersuchungen über Atherosklerose. Über bindegewebige Intimaverdickungen und spontane Lipidose der Aorta und anderer Organe bei Hunden. Zieglers Beiträge: vide Beitr. path. Anat. *88:* 241–314 (1932).

IX. Illustrations

Page 103

Fig. 1. Aorta, descending thoracic segment, dog. Medial smooth muscle cells are shown in cross section. Two layers of smooth muscle cells are shown with associated elastic fibers (pale staining homogeneous fibers). The space between the lamellae of smooth muscle and elastin fibers contains numerous collagen fibers and small fibers of elastin. All cells seen are smooth muscle. The principal cytoplasmic organelle in the smooth muscle cells is myofilaments which, at this low magnification, imparts a ground-glass appearance to the cytoplasm. Numerous small areas of electron density are apparent among the myofilaments and along the plasma membranes. Approximately × 3,200. (Reproduced with permission from Geer, J. C. and Guidry, M. A.: Experimental canine atherosclerosis, chapt. 22; in Roberts and Straus Comparative atherosclerosis. Hoeber, Evanston/Harper & Row London 1965.)

Page 104

Fig. 2. Aorta, descending thoracic segment, 16-year-old male. Smooth muscle cell. Elastic fibers in the interstitial along the left margin of the micrograph are electron-lucid. Adjacent to the plasma membrane of the smooth muscle cell, there is electron-dense basement membrane. Micropinocytotic vesicles are present in the plasma membrane of the cell. Mitochondria and endoplasmic reticulum are present primarily in the region of the nucleus, especially at the upper margin of the nucleus. The remainder of the cytoplasm contains myofilaments among which there are numerous areas of density in which the filaments converge. At the lower margin of the nucleus, there is a dense inclusion consisting of homogeneous areas and dense granular material, lipofuscin pigment. × 14,000.

Page 105

Fig. 3. Coronary artery, left anterior descending branch, male, age 20 years. This is a longitudinal section. The medial smooth muscle cells appear in cross section, spiral orientation. The intimal smooth muscle cells are arranged longitudinally. Elastic fibers appear black in the micrograph. The internal elastic membrane is not present. The junction of intima and media is indistinct and can be localized only by observing the orientation of the muscle cells. This is a typical musculo-elastic intima, diffuse intimal thickening. The subendothelial connective tissue layer is well developed. Phosphotungstic acid-hematoxylin stain. Approximately × 250. (Reproduced with permission from Robertson, W. B.; Geer, J. C.; Strong, J. P., and McGill, H. C., jr.: The fate of the fatty streak. Exp. molec. Path. (suppl.) *1:* 28–39, 1963.)

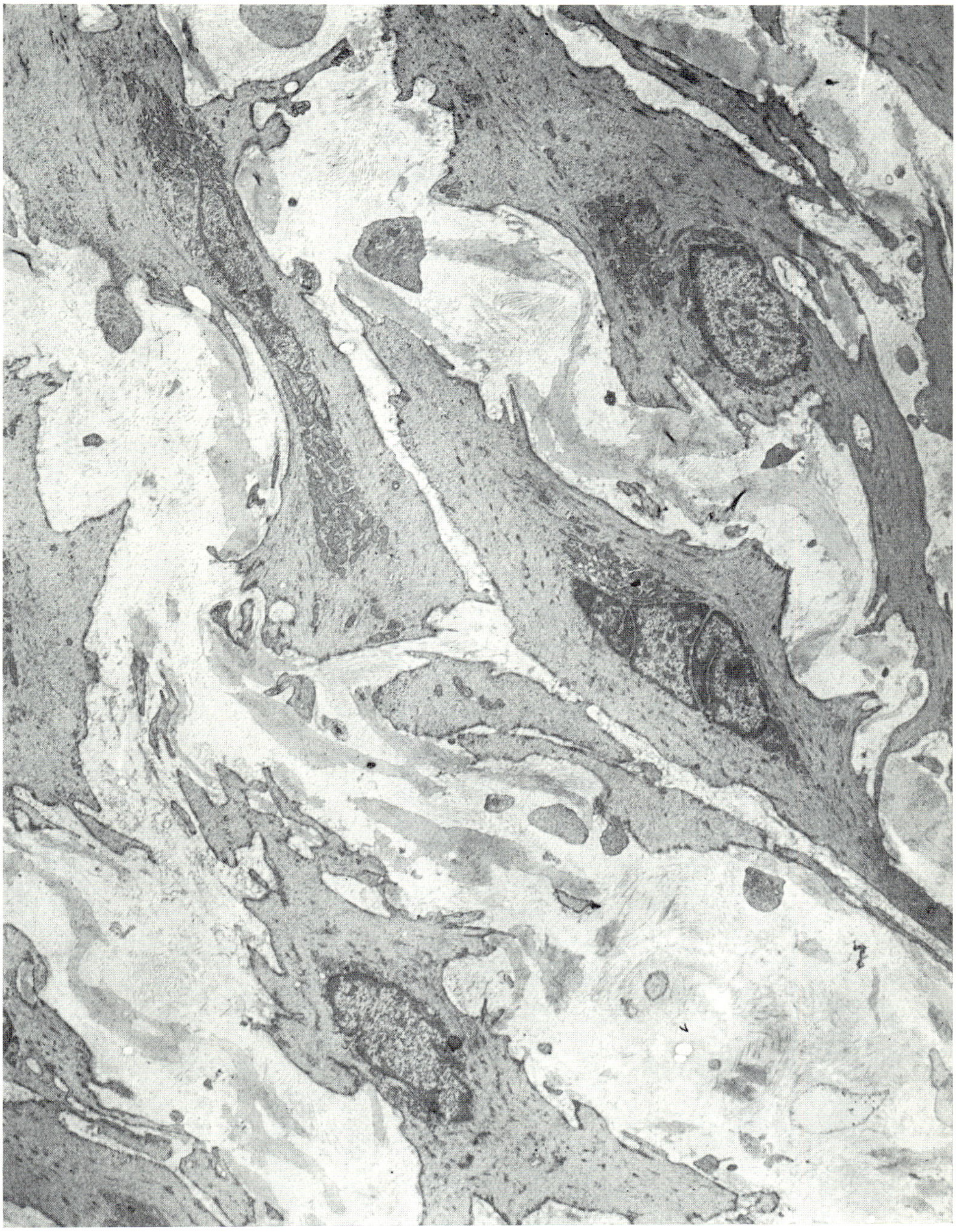

1

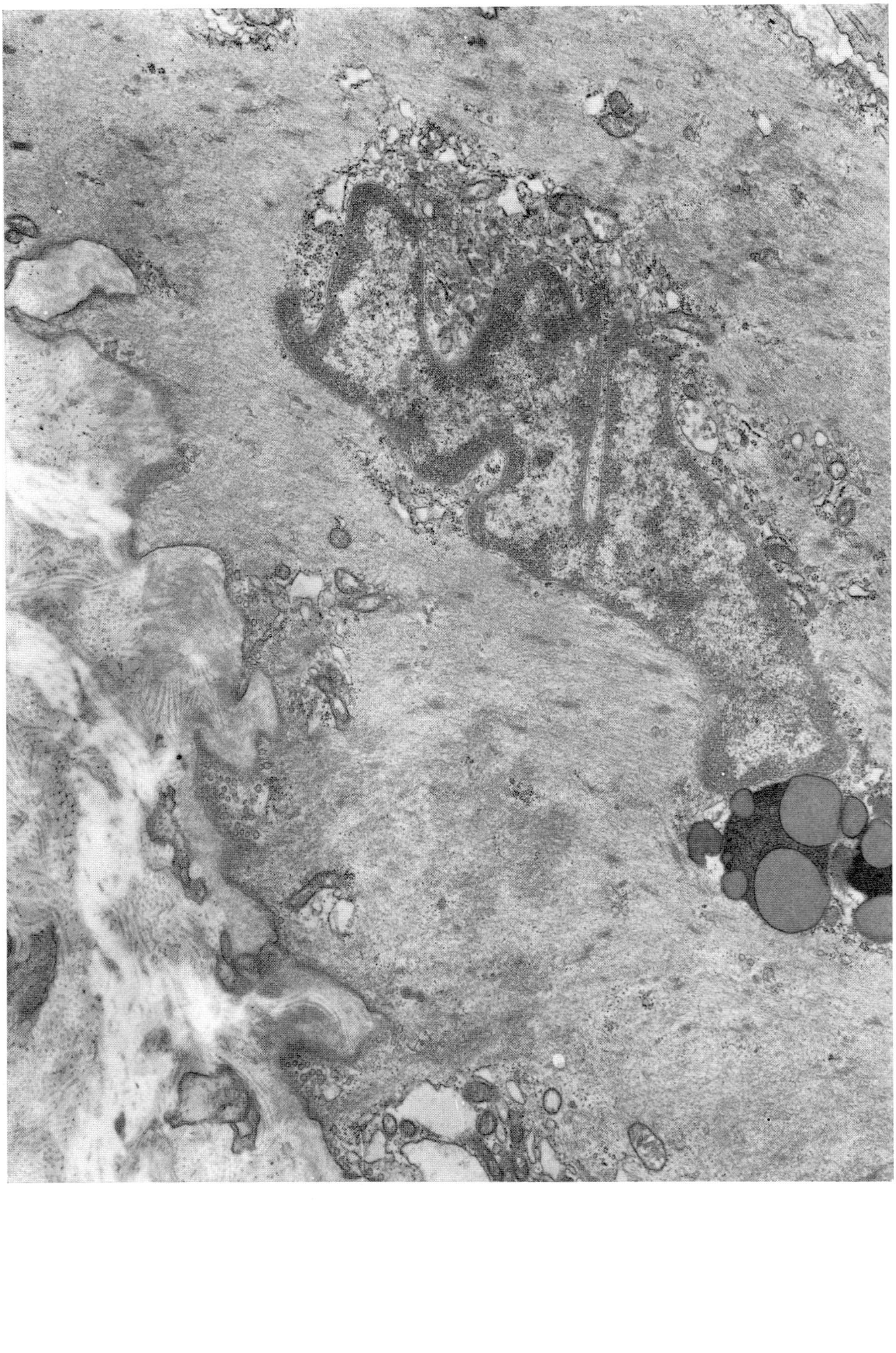

2

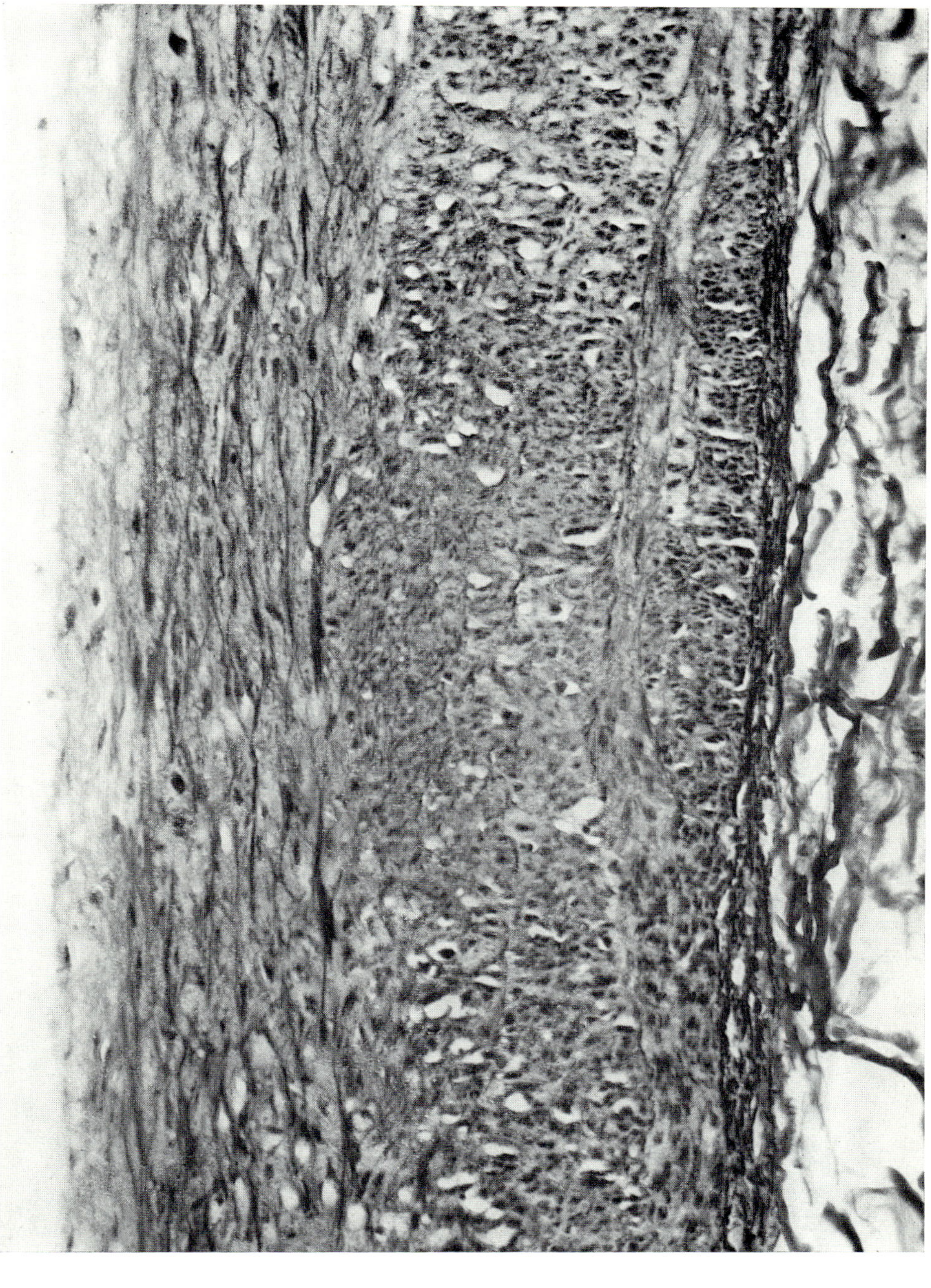

3

Page 107

Fig. 4a. Thoracic aorta, adolescent. The internal elastic membrane appears black in the micrograph because of lipid encrustation. The intima is slightly thickened, note right half of micrograph. Oil-red-O-hematoxylin stain. Approximately ×150. *b* Abdominal aorta, adolescent. Elastic fibers near the media and, to a lesser degree, in the intima appear black in the micrograph because of lipid encrustation. The intima is considerably and more diffusely thickened in the abdominal segment of the aorta than in the thoracic segment; compare to a. Oil-red O hematoxylin stain. Approximately ×150.

Page 108

Fig. 5. Coronary artery, left anterior descending branch, male adolescent. Portions of the internal elastic membrane are present. The intima shows musculo-elastic thickening. On the lumen surface of the intima, there is a thin layer of fibrin, black in the micrograph, a mural thrombus. Phosphotungstic acid-hematoxylin stain. Approximately ×275.

Page 109

Fig. 6a. Coronary artery, left anterior descending branch, male, age 25 years. This is a longitudinal section of the artery like that seen in figures 3 and 4, medial cells are cut in cross section and intimal cells longitudinally. Numerous intimal cells have lipid in their cytoplasm, black in the micrograph. Oil-red-O-hematoxylin stain. Approximately ×250. (Reproduced with permission from ROBERTSON, W. B.; GEER, J. C.; STRONG, J. P., and MCGILL, H. C., jr.: The fate of the fatty streak. Exp. molec. Path. (suppl.) *1:* 28–39, 1963.) *b* Coronary artery intima, plastic embedded section. Note large, round foam cells in intima near left margin of the micrograph. Approximately ×430.

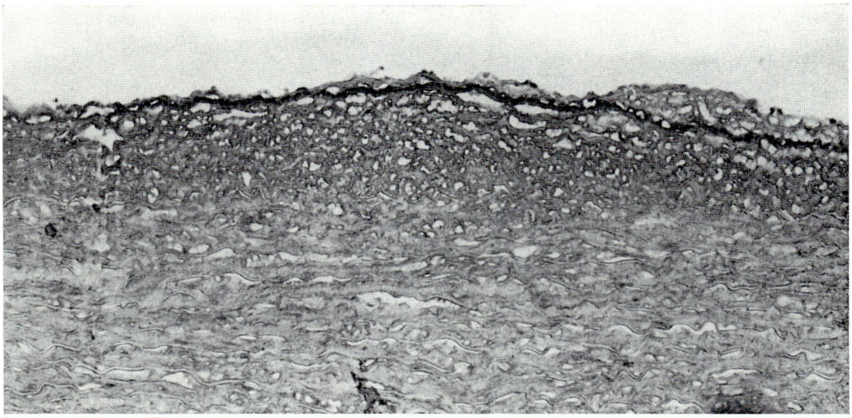

4a

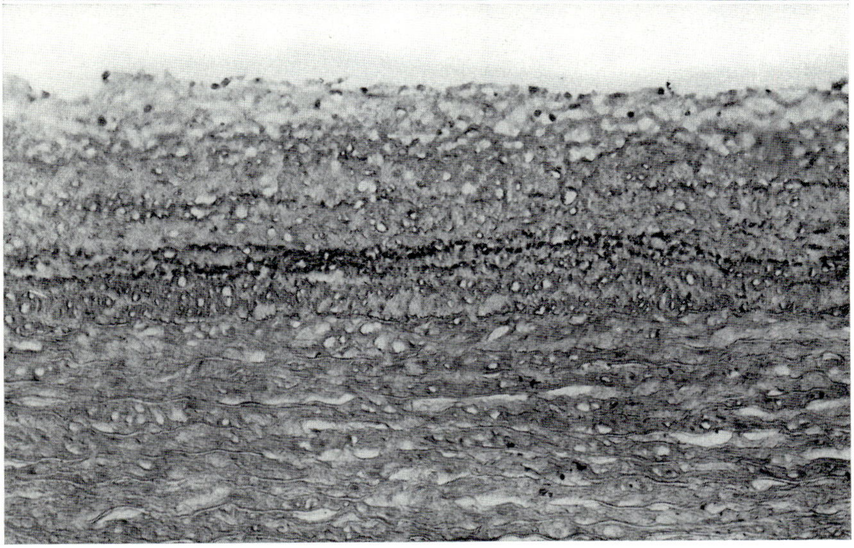

4b

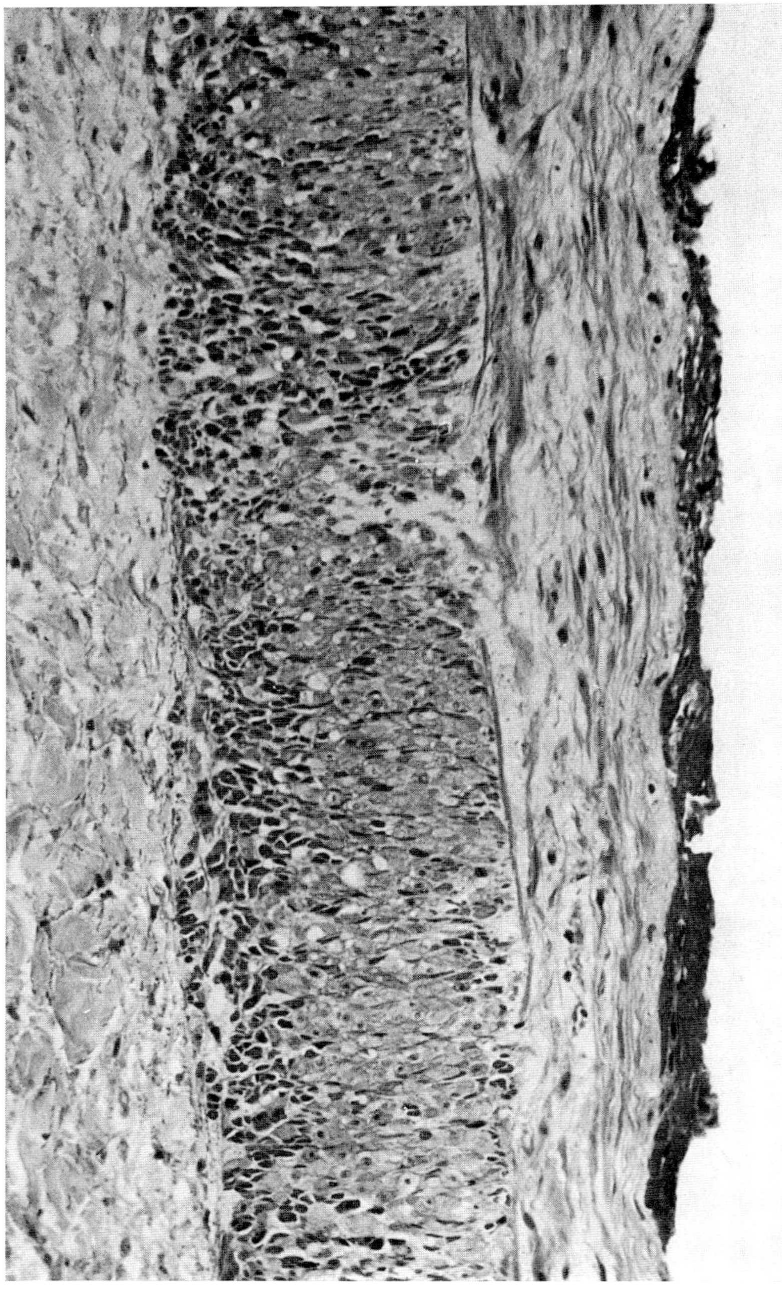

5

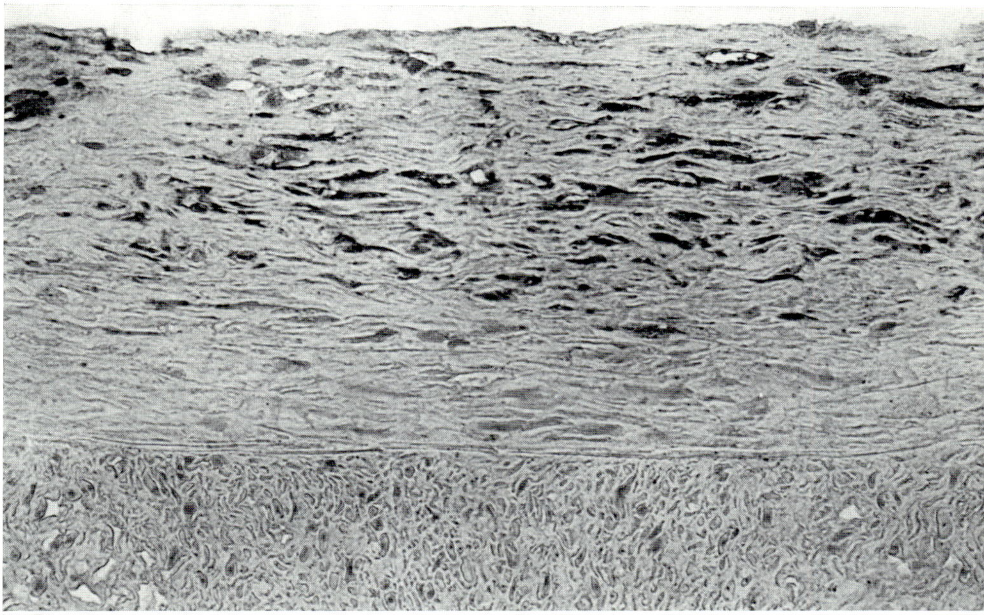
6a

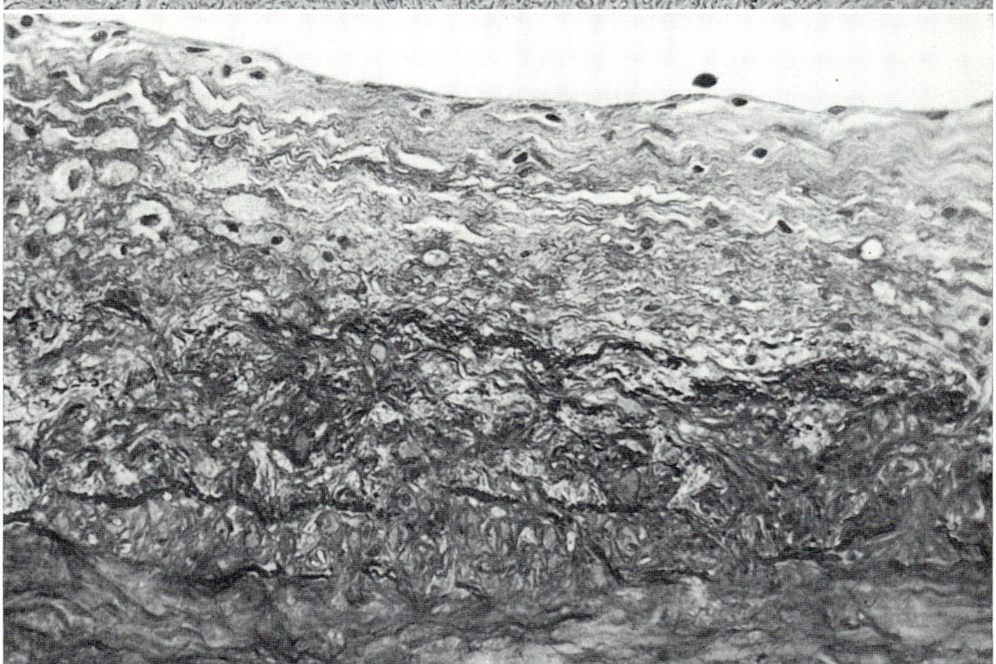
6b

Page 111

Fig. 7. Aorta, descending thoracic segment, fatty streak lesion, male, age 16 years. The endothelial cell depicted overlies a fatty streak. This endothelial cell has more numerous cytoplasmic organelles (mitochondria, endoplasmic reticulum, vacuoles, myelin-like figures, and Golgi membranes) than endothelium overlying normal intima. Basement membrane relation to the intimal surface of the cell is distorted, probably because of contraction. Thin filaments are present in the cytoplasm adjacent to the nucleus. Electron-dense granular-appearing material is present in the interstitial tissue of the intima. A portion of a cell is present at the lower right margin of the micrograph in which-electron dense material is contained that is similar in appearance to that in the interstitial tissue. Approximately × 18,750. (Reproduced with permission from GEER, J. C.: Fine structure of human aortic intimal thickening and fatty streaks. Lab. Invest. *14:* 1764–1783, 1965.)

Page 112

Fig. 8. Aorta, descending thoracic segment, normal gross appearance, male, age 2 ½ months. Stellate-shaped cell in intima of uncertain identification. There is very little cytoplasm in the region of the nucleus, and the cytoplasm extends from the cell body with thin processes containing granular endoplasmic reticulum. Thin filaments are present in the cytoplasm at the upper margin of the nucleus and in the cytoplasmic extension toward the right margin of the micrograph. There are small segments of basement membrane associated with the body of the cell. Elastic fibers appear electron-lucid in the interstitial tissue; many have a mantle of microfilaments around them. Abundant collagen fibers are present in the interstitial tissue. At the upper and lower right corners of the micrograph, there are membrane-bound bodies containing faint filaments or granular material; these are 'ghost bodies'. Approximately × 8,700. (Reproduced with permission from GEER, J. C.: Fine structure of human aortic intimal thickening and fatty streaks. Lab. Invest. *14:* 1764–1783, 1965.)

Page 113

Fig. 9. Aorta, descending thoracic segment, fatty streak lesion, male, age 16 years. The cell in the center of the micrograph is irregular in shape, with numerous cytoplasmic organelles in the perinuclear region or cell body and thin extension of the cytoplasm into the surrounding interstitial tissue. The cytoplasmic extensions are thinner and longer than those usually found in smooth muscle cells; however, this cell has filaments in the cytoplasm that appear to be myofilaments and has a basement membrane associated with the plasma membrane in many areas. In addition to elastic fibers and collagen fibrils in the interstitial tissue, there are electron-dense granular bodies. A portion of smooth muscle cytoplasm at the right margin of the micrograph has a lipid inclusion. Approximately × 12,500. (Reproduced with permission from GEER, J. C. and MCGILL, H. C., jr.: The evolution of the fatty streak, chapt. 2; in BREST and MOYER Atherosclerotic vascular disease. Appleton-Century-Crofts, New York 1967.)

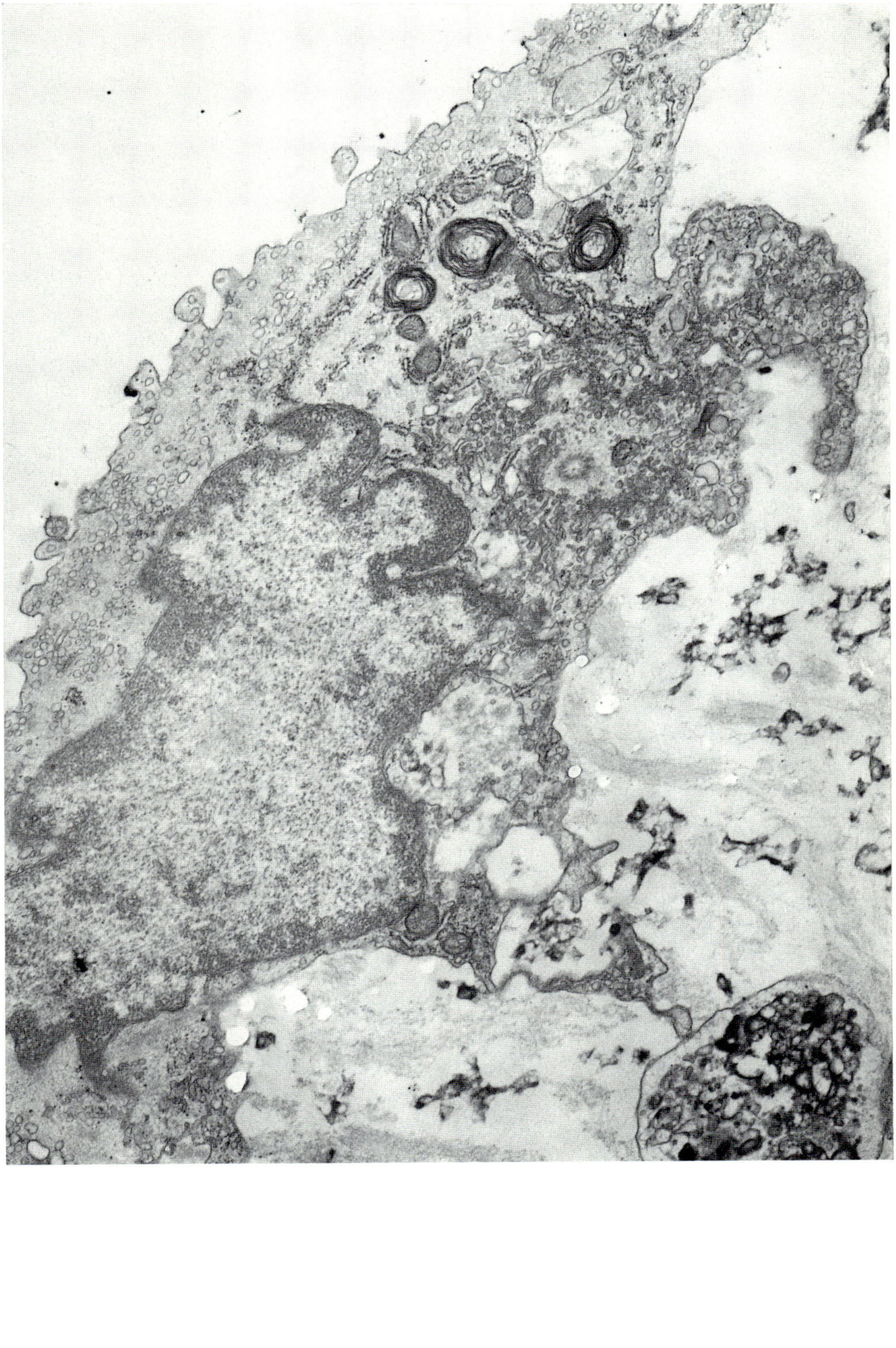

7

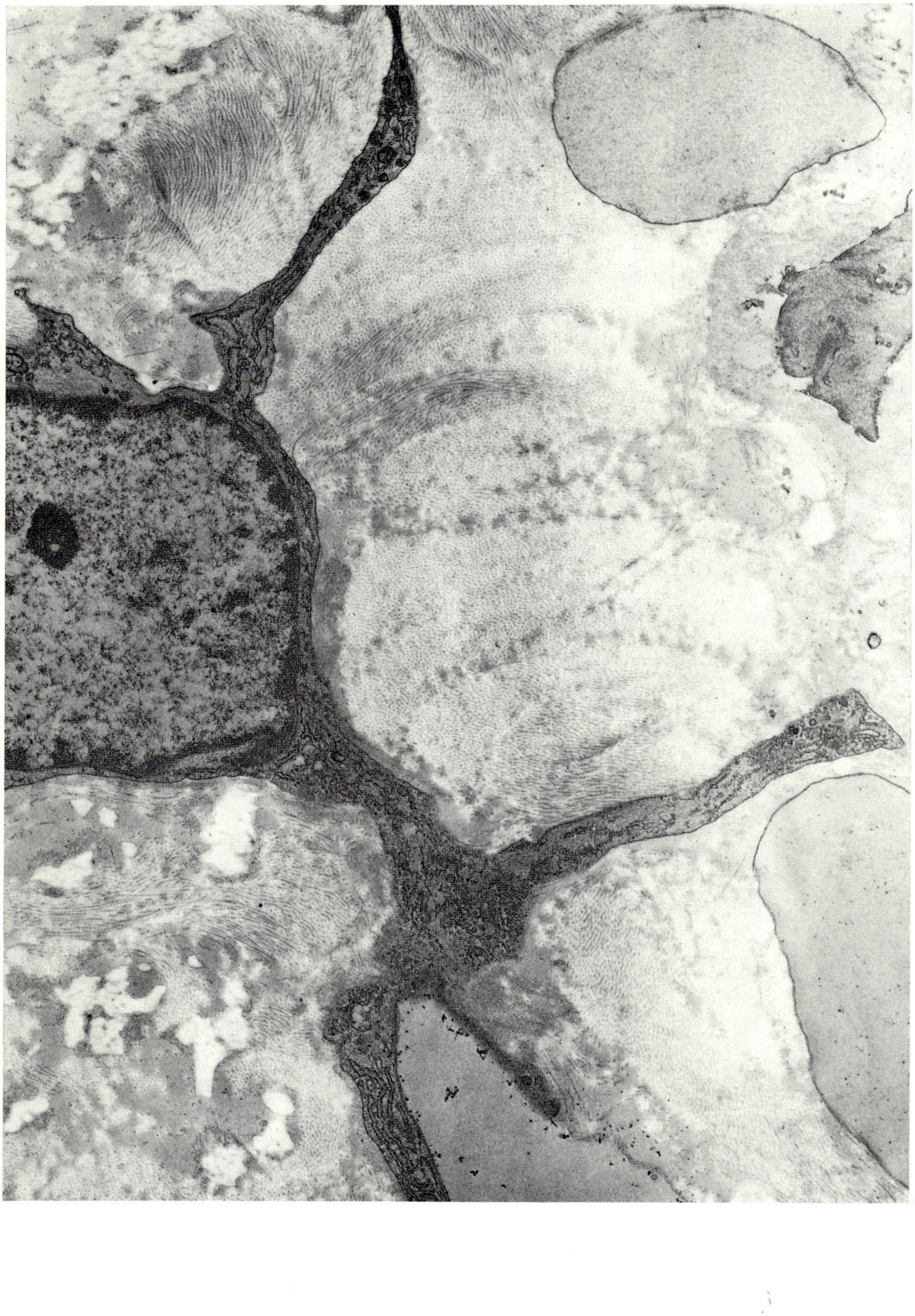

8

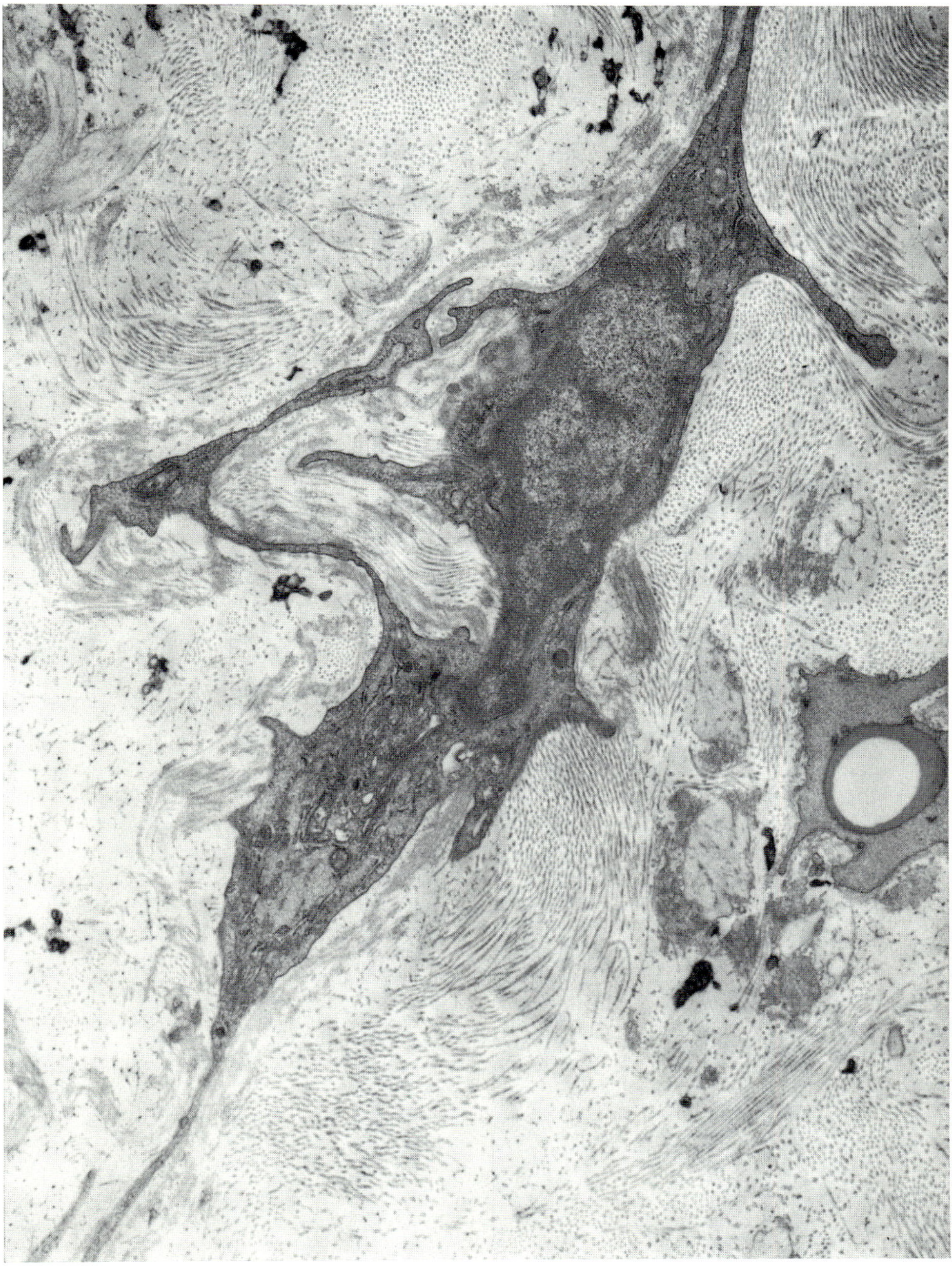

9

Page 115

Fig. 10. Aorta, descending thoracic segment, fatty streak lesion, male, age 24 years. The larger cell in the center of the micrograph is similar to that in figure 9, except for more abundant profiles of granular endoplasmic reticulum in the cytoplasm and a complete limiting basement membrane. A lipid inclusion is present in the cytoplasm at the right margin of the micrograph. The cell in the lower portion of the micrograph has no limiting basement membrane and contains few cytoplasmic organelles, except free ribonucleoprotein granules. This cell resembles a blood monocyte or lymphocyte. Note the electron-dense granular material in the interstitial space at the left margin of the micrograph. Approximately × 18,700. (Reproduced with permission from GEER, J. C. and MCGILL, H. C., jr.: The evolution of the fatty streak, chapt. 2; in BREST and MOYER Atherosclerotic vascular disease. Appleton-Century-Crofts, New York 1967.)

Page 116

Fig. 11. Aorta, descending thoracic segment, fatty streak lesion, male, age 16 years. Irregularly shaped cell of uncertain identity in aortic intima. This cell has no recognizable basement membrane. There are numerous micropinocytotic vesicles along the plasma membrane. The cytoplasm contains rather numerous cisternae of granular endoplasmic reticulum in which a flocculent-appearing material is visible. Fine filaments are present in the cytoplasm. No dense areas are seen among the filaments like those in typical smooth muscle cells. Approximately × 14,700.

Page 117

Fig. 12. Aorta, descending thoracic segment, fatty streak lesion, male, age 24 years. The cell in the center of the micrograph and the portions of cells at the upper and lower margins are typical smooth muscle cells with a limiting basement membrane, numerous micropinocytotic vesicles along the plasma membrane, and abundant myofilaments in the cytoplasm. The middle cell and the portion of a cell at the lower margin of the micrograph contain cytoplasmic lipid inclusions. These inclusions have a scalloped margin and are homogeneous in appearance. There is no appreciable increase in the number of mitochondria or profiles of endoplasmic reticulum in the center cell over that expected in a smooth muscle cell not containing lipid inclusions. Note the electron-dense granular material in the extracellular space. Approximately × 16,000. (Reproduced with permission from GEER, J. C. and GUIDRY, M. A.: Cholesteryl ester composition and morphology of human normal intima and fatty streaks. Exp. molec. Path. *3:* 485–499, 1964.)

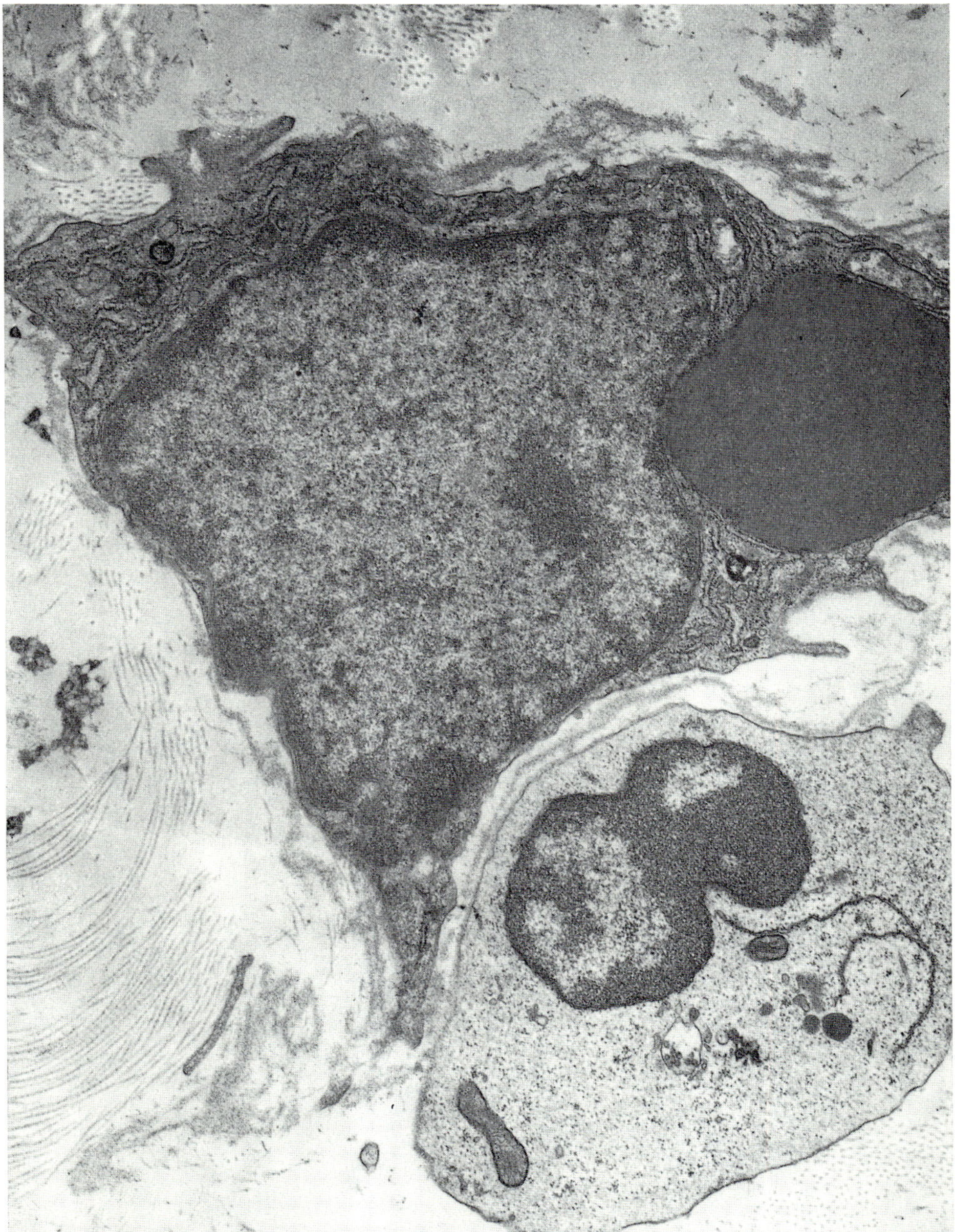

10

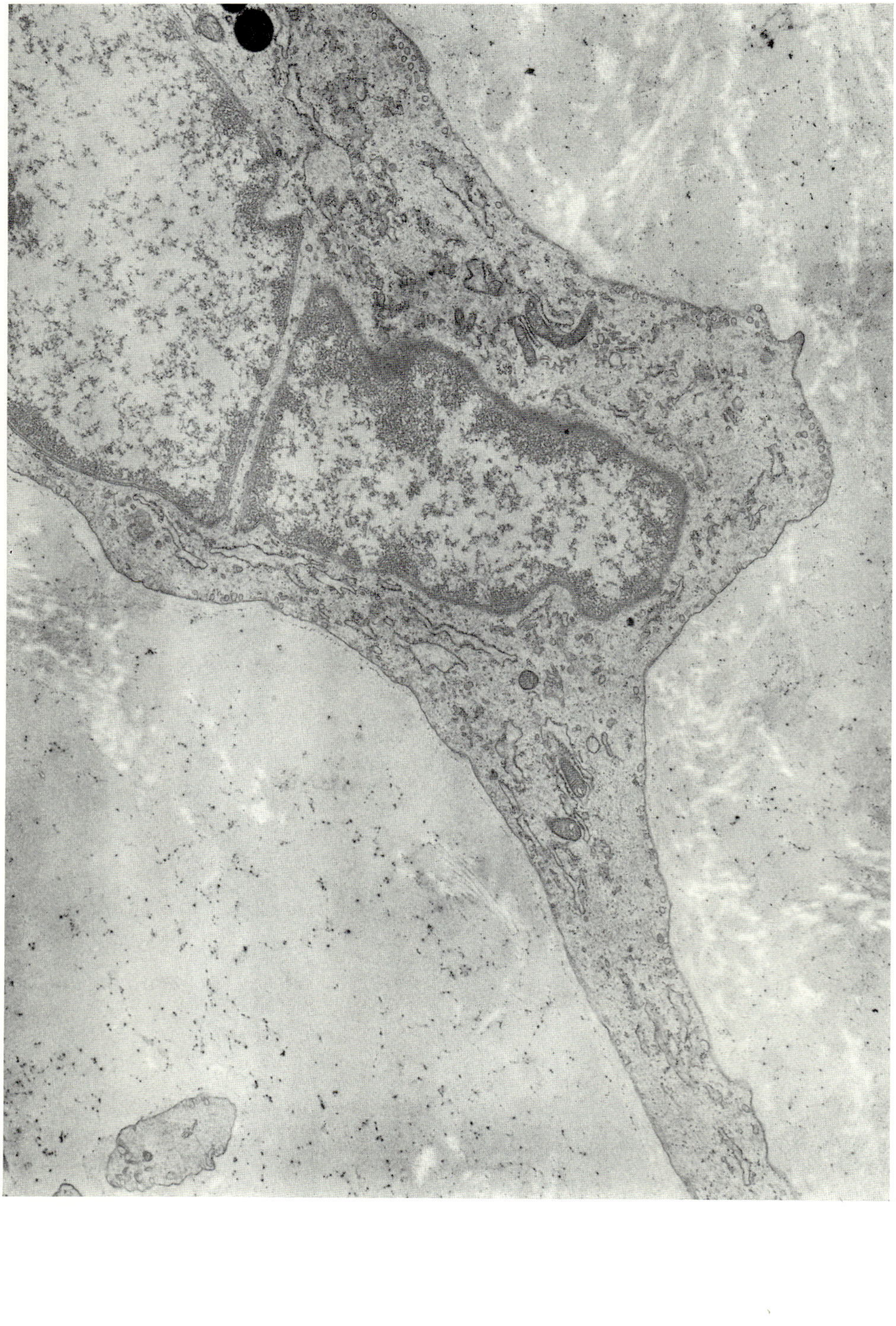

11

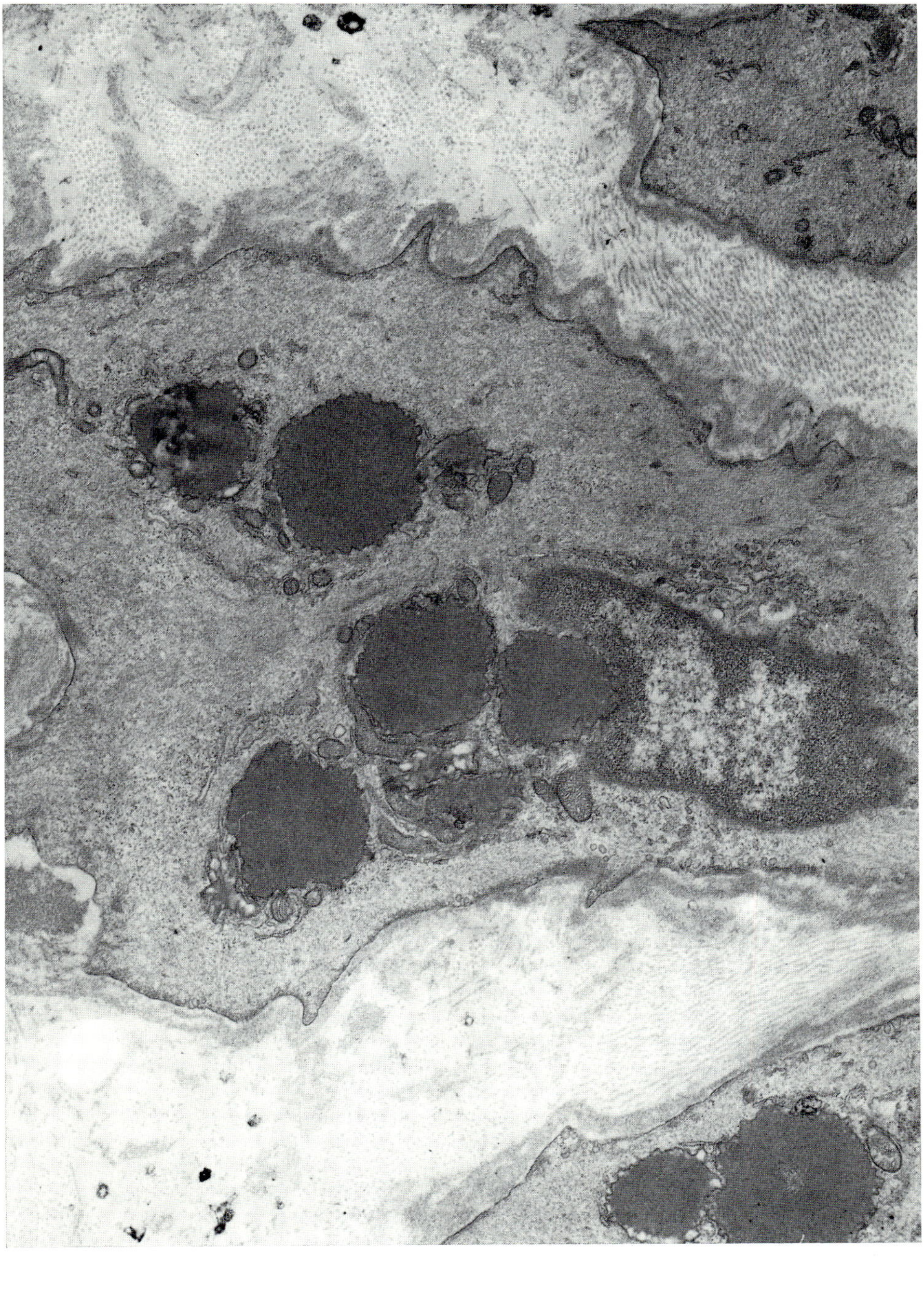

12

Page 119

Fig. 13. Aorta, descending thoracic segment, fatty streak lesion, male, age 16 years. This smooth muscle cell with one lipid inclusion in the cytoplasm shows a marked increase in the number of mitochondria and profiles of endoplasmic reticulum over that seen in normal smooth muscle cells. The lipid inclusion has a slightly irregular margin and is composed of a peripheral rim of moderately electron-dense homogenous material and a central electron-lucid zone. Myofilaments are present in the region of the plasma membrane, and the central area of the cell is occupied primarily by other cytoplasmic organelles. Note the electron-dense granular material in the interstitial space at the lower right corner of the micrograph. Approximately × 14,900.

Page 120

Fig. 14. Aorta, descending thoracic segment, fatty streak lesion, male, age 24 years. Smooth muscle cells with numerous lipid inclusions in their cytoplasm. Neither cell shows any appreciable increase in the number of mitochondria or profiles of endoplasmic reticulum over that seen in normal smooth muscle. Note the difference in morphology of the lipid inclusions in these cells from those in figures 12 and 13. Many of the inclusions in this micrograph show an apparent shrinkage of the lipid from the margin of the inclusion, tending to impart a 'spoked-wheel' appearance. There is abundant electron-dense granular material in the interstitial space intermingled with less electron-dense flocculo-fibrillar material at the top and bottom of the micrograph. Approximately × 14,700. (Reproduced with permission from Geer, J. C. and Guidry, M. A.: Cholesteryl ester composition and morphology of human normal intima and fatty streaks. Exp. molec. Path. *3:* 485–499, 1963.)

Page 121

Fig. 15. Aorta, descending thoracic segment, fatty streak lesion, male, age 16 years. The smooth muscle cell at the left side of the micrograph shows lipid inclusions in the cytoplasm, associated with an increased number of mitochondria and profiles of endoplasmic reticulum. This cell does not show a complete limiting basement membrane. The cell to the right of the smooth muscle cell has ovoid-shaped mitochondria in contrast to the elongated ones in the smooth muscle cell and few other cytoplasmic organelles – profiles of agranular endoplasmic reticulum and free ribonucleoprotein particles. This cell has cytoplasmic pseudopodial extensions, is similar to that in figure 10, and resembles a blood monocyte or lymphocyte. Note the large amount of electron-dense granular material in the interstitial space in the lower right corner of the micrograph. Approximately × 13,800. (Reproduced with permission from Geer, J. C. and McGill, H. C., jr.: The evolution of the fatty streak, chapt. 2; in Brest and Moyer Atherosclerotic vascular disease. Appleton-Century-Crofts, New York 1967.)

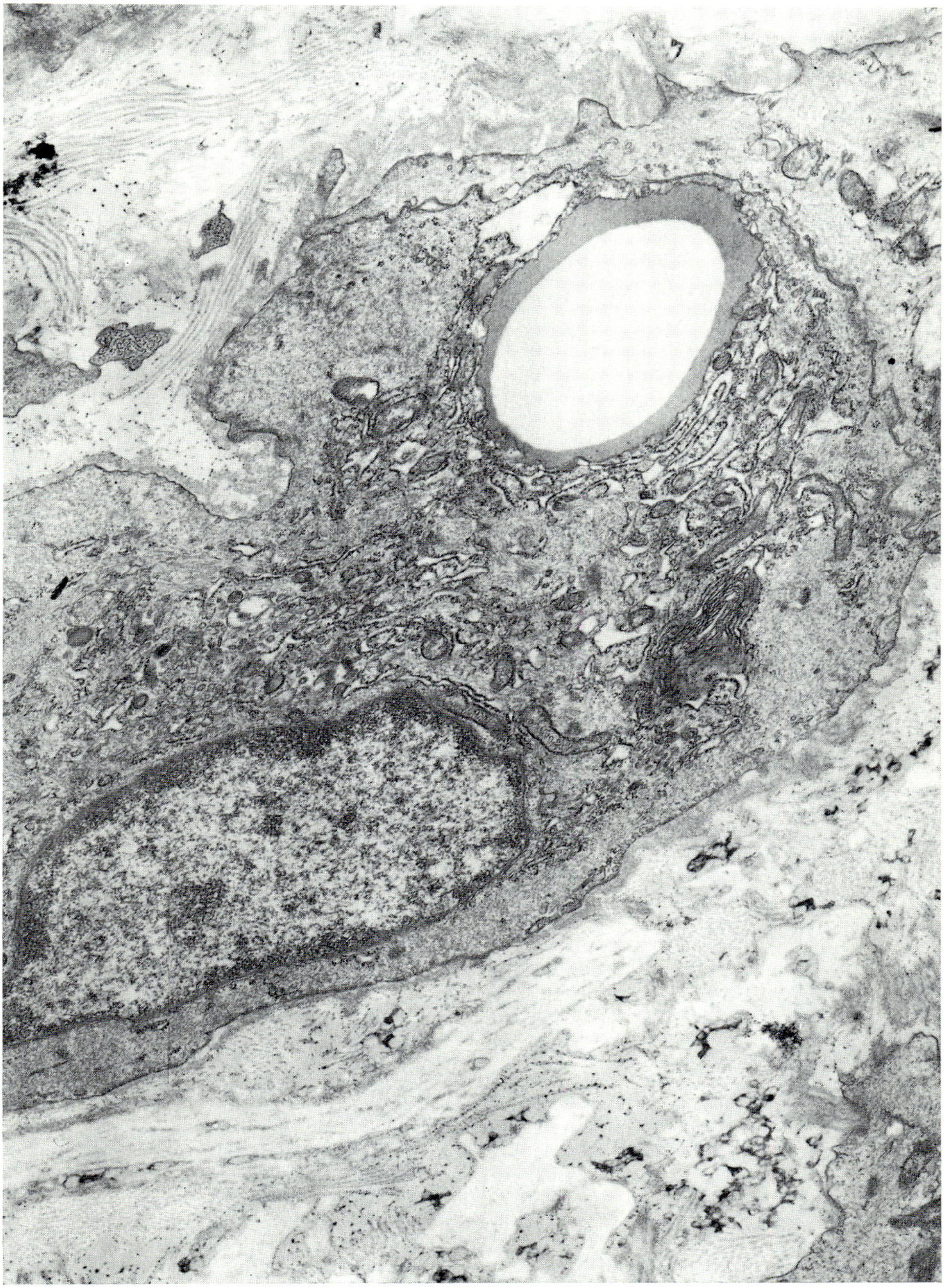

13

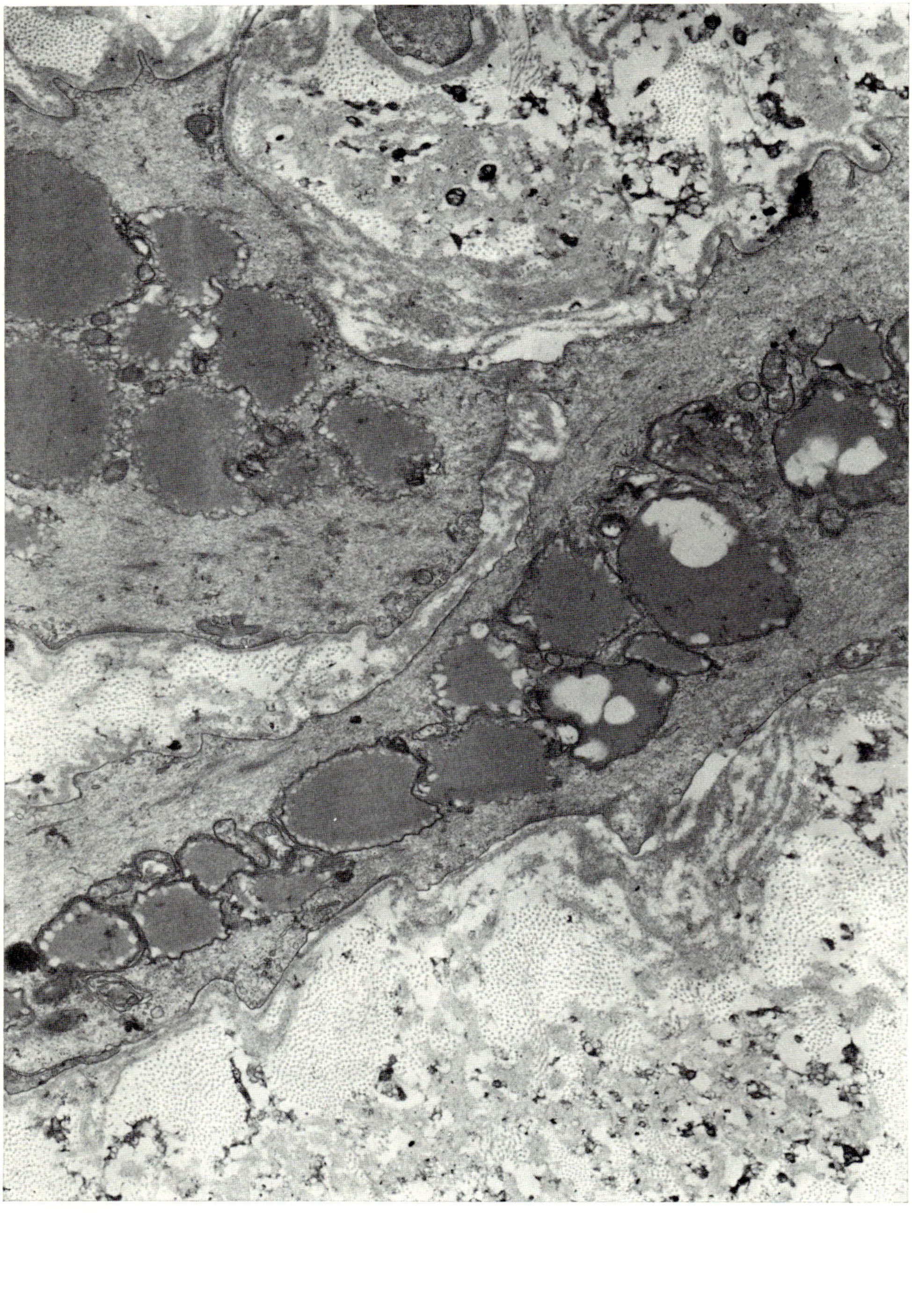

14

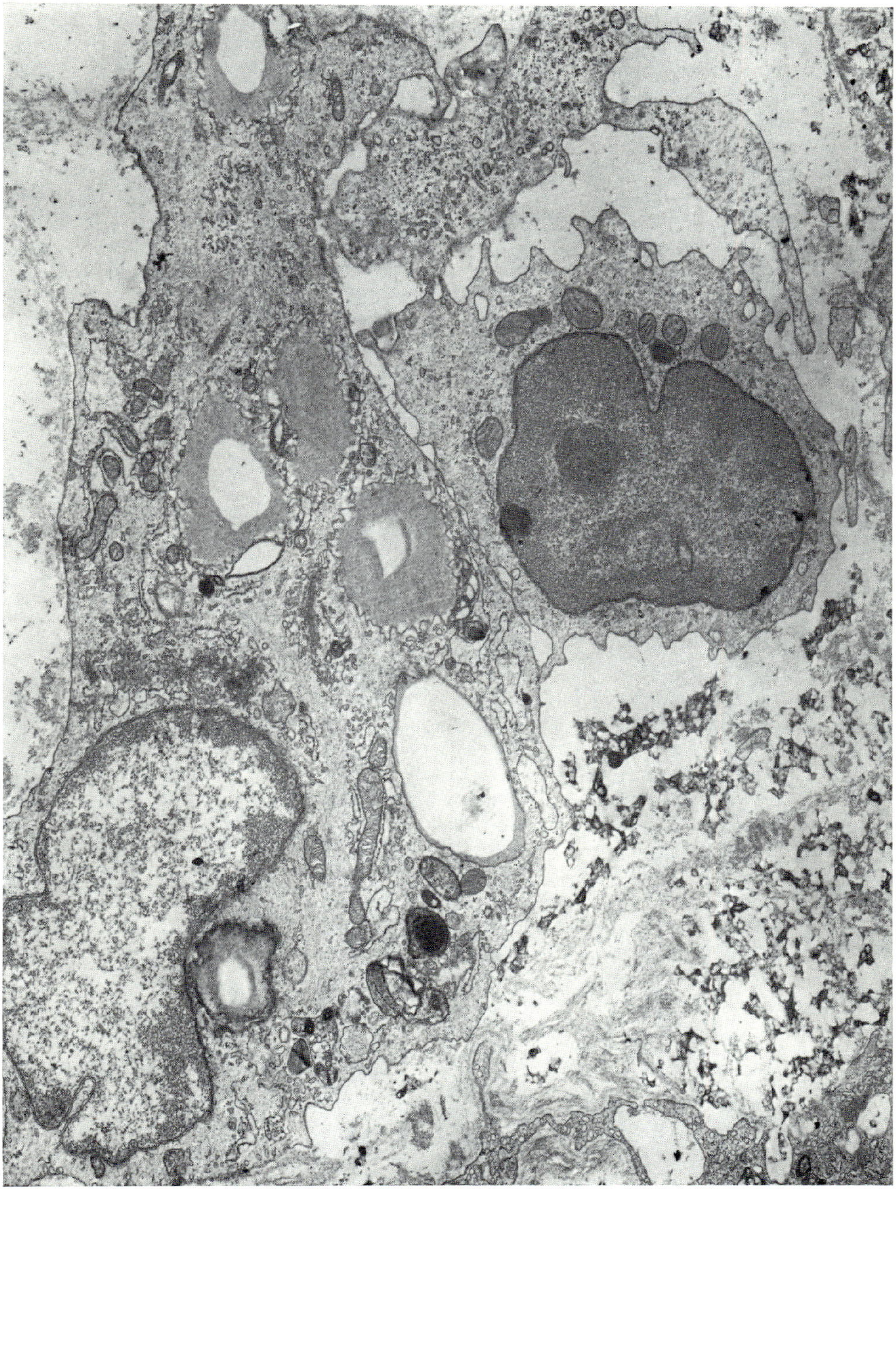

15

Page 123

Fig. 16. Aorta, descending thoracic segment, fatty streak lesion, male, age 24 years. This cell resembling a blood monocyte or lymphocyte is similar to those in figures 10 and 15, except for the presence of more numerous profiles of agranular endoplasmic reticulum. These cells are present in all human fatty streak lesions and usually are found near the endothelium. Approximately × 14,700.

Page 124

Fig. 17. Aorta, descending thoracic segment, fatty streak lesion, male age 24 years. This cell has none of the morphological features that are used to identify smooth muscle. The cell resembles those shown in figures 10, 15, and 16, except for a marked increase in the number of cytoplasmic organelles and the presence of lipid inclusions in the cytoplasm. The finding of cells such as this has suggested to some observers that those cells resembling blood monocytes or lymphocytes accumulate lipid in the intima and become the large ovoid foam cell. Note the electron-dense material in the interstitial space. This cell shows no morphological evidence of phagocytosis of the extracellular dense material. Approximately × 15 400. (Reproduced with permission from GEER J. C.: Fine structure of human aortic intimal thickening and fatty streaks. Lab. Invest. *14:* 1764–1783 1965.)

Page 125

Fig. 18. Aorta descending thoracic segment, fatty streak lesion, male, age 21 years. The cell at the top of the micrograph is typical smooth muscle with lipid inclusions in the cytoplasm. The cell in the lower portion of the micrograph has none of the morphological features that are used to identify smooth muscle. The identity or origin of this cell is unknown. There are four typical lipid inclusions in the cytoplasm resembling those in the smooth muscle cell. In addition there are numerous vacuoles in the cytoplasm containing electron-dense granular material similar to that observed in the interstitial tissue in figures 7, 9, 10, 12–16, 20, 23, 25, 26. Vacuoles such as these have suggested to some that this cell is phagocytosing the electron-dense granular material from the extracellular space. Similar vacuoles are found in cells showing obvious degenerative changes suggesting that such vacuoles represent cytoplasmic degeneration. The cell in this micrograph has no other evidence suggesting degeneration (compare with fig. 24). Note the forming elastic elements (moderately electron-dense) in the interstitial space. Approximately × 20 000.

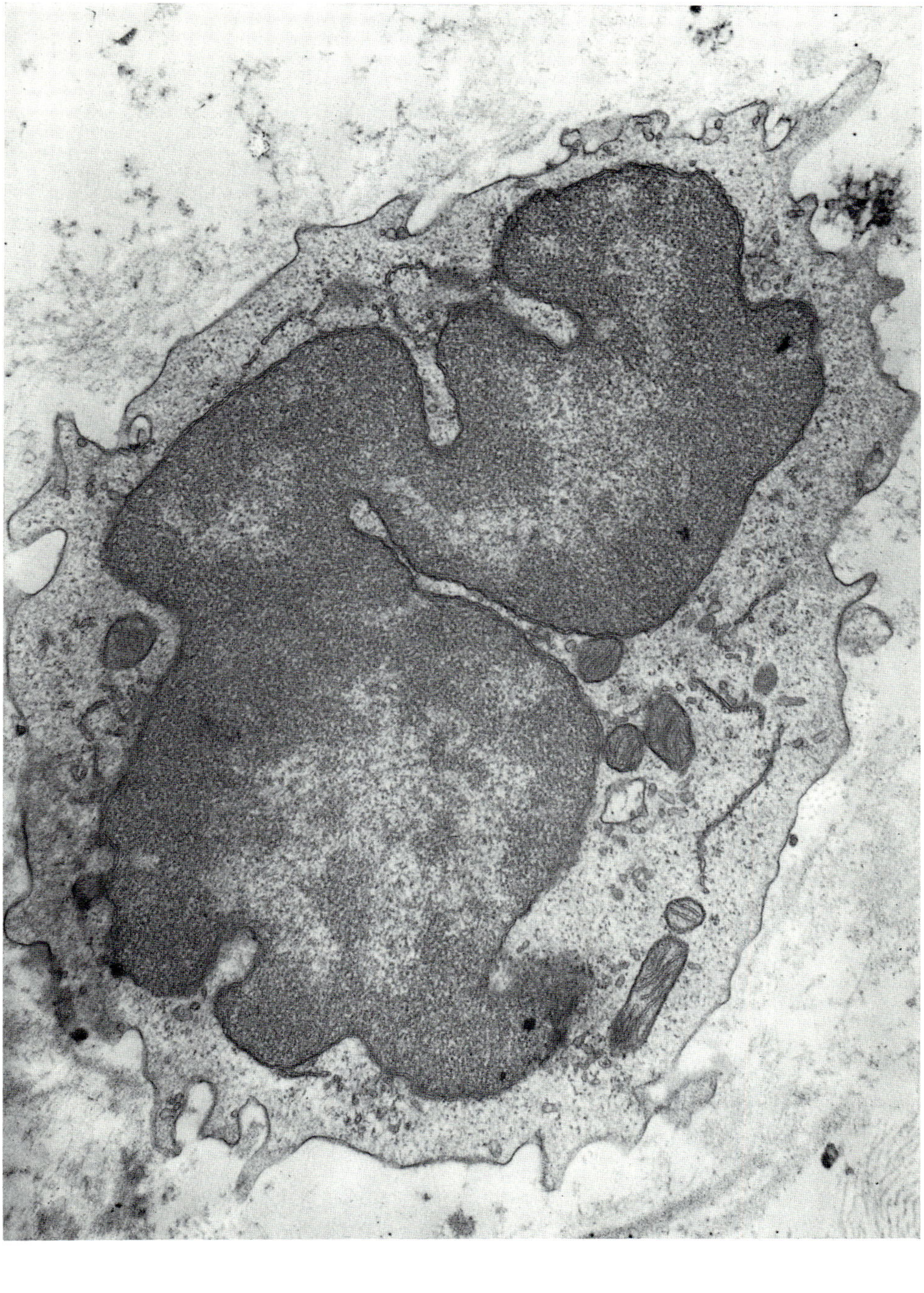

16

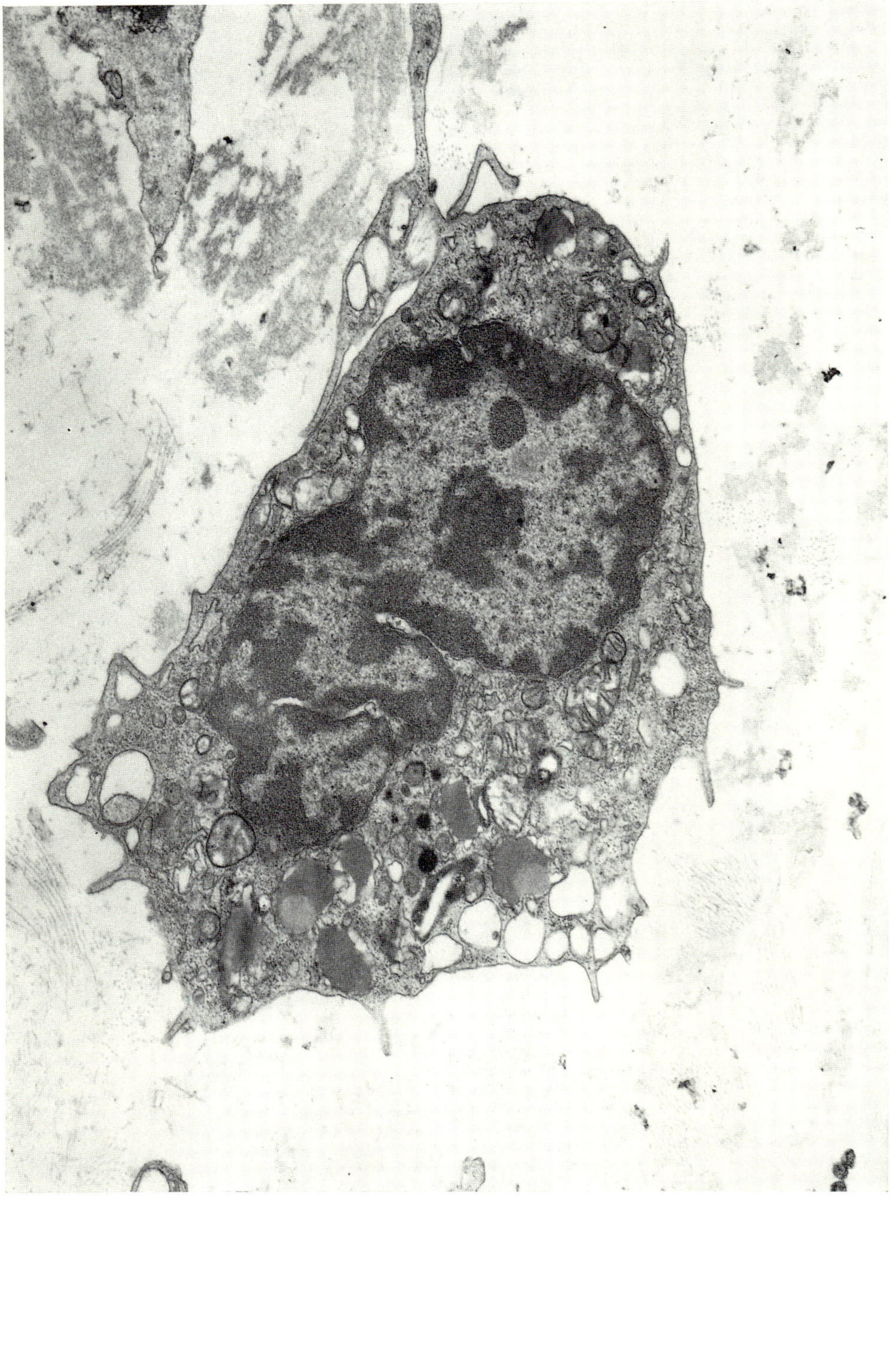

17

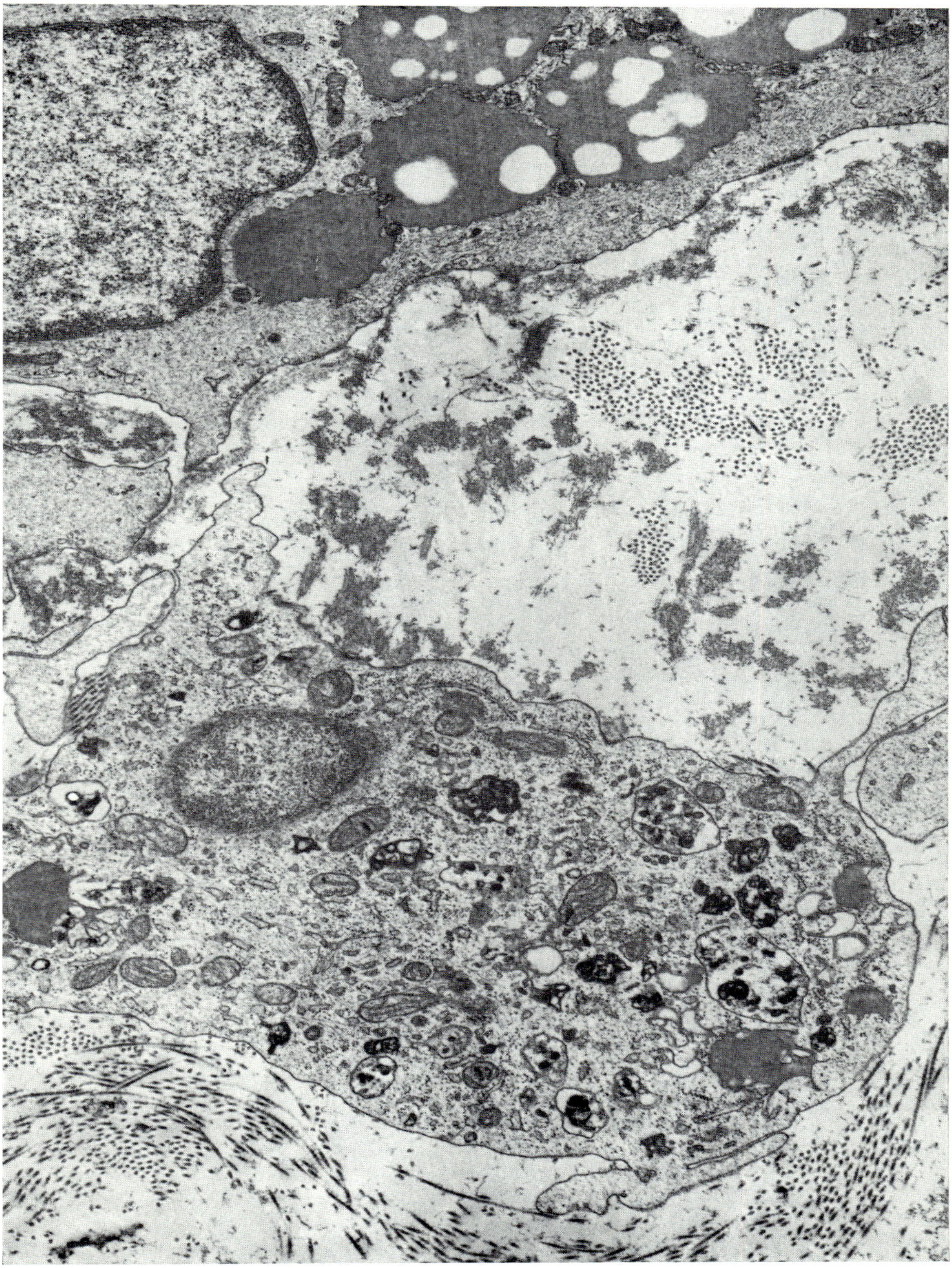

18

Page 127

Fig. 19. Aorta, rabbit fed diet with cholesterol added. Large foam cell containing many morphological forms of cytoplasmic inclusions resting immediately adjacent to a thin rim of aortic endothelium. Note the junctions of endothelial cells in the upper and lower portions of the micrograph (arrows). Approximately × 10 000.

Page 128

Fig. 20. Aorta, serial section of figure 19. Note that the cell is penetrating the endothelium through and not between endothelial cells. The direction in which this cell is moving cannot be determined in static micrographs. Approximately × 10 000.

Page 129

Fig. 21. Aorta, descending thoracic segment, fatty streak lesion, male, age 24 years. This micrograph contrasts the appearance of a myogenic foam cell (left) and large ovoid foam cell (right). The myogenic foam cell has basement membrane electron-dense cytoplasmic lipid inclusions, and a thin margin of myofilaments along the plasma membrane. The ovoid cell, in contrast, has no basement membrane, less dense lipid inclusions in addition to a variety of other and unidentified inclusions, and no myofilaments. There is electron-dense granular material in the extracellular space. Approximately × 5 000.

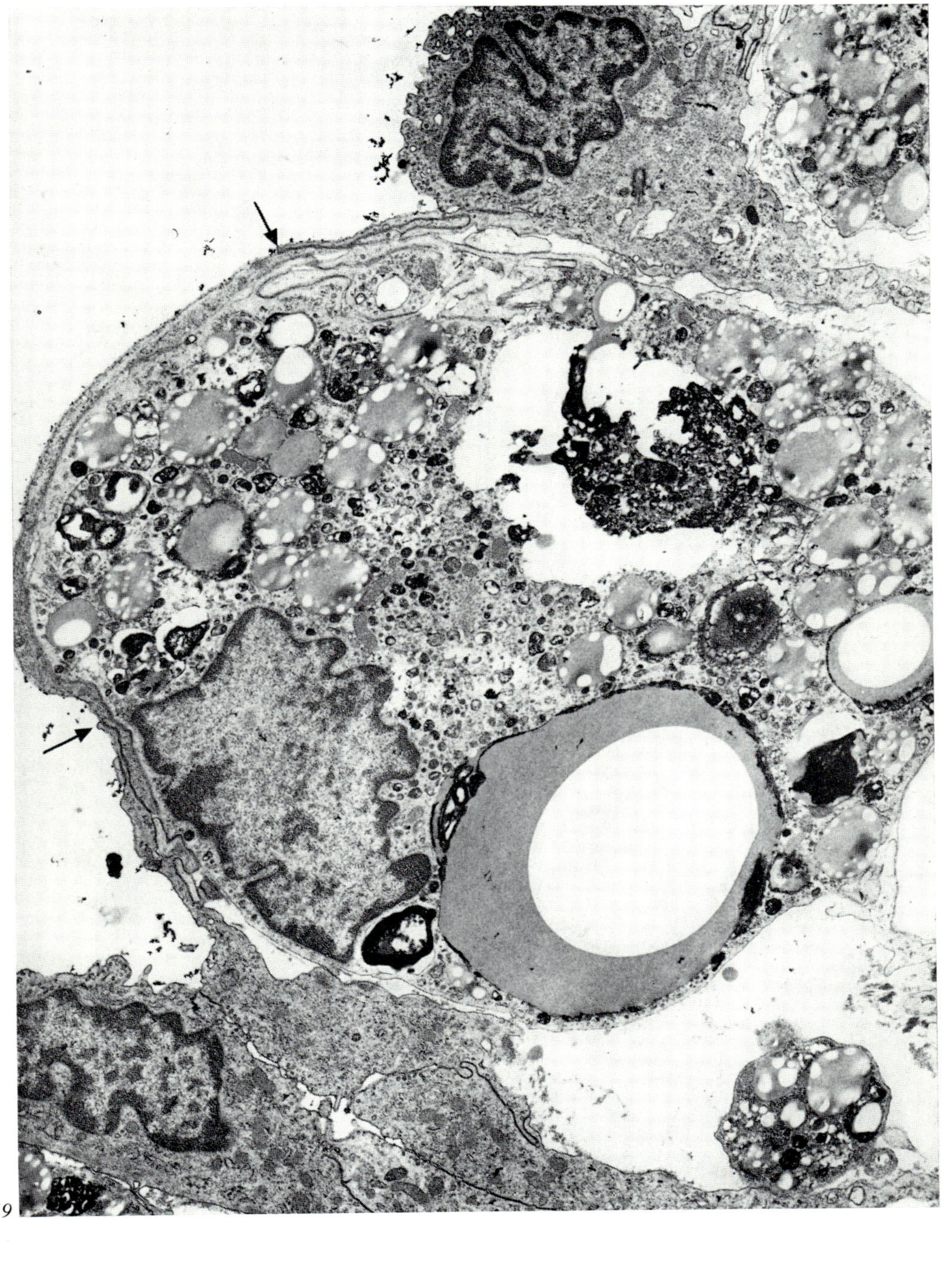

19

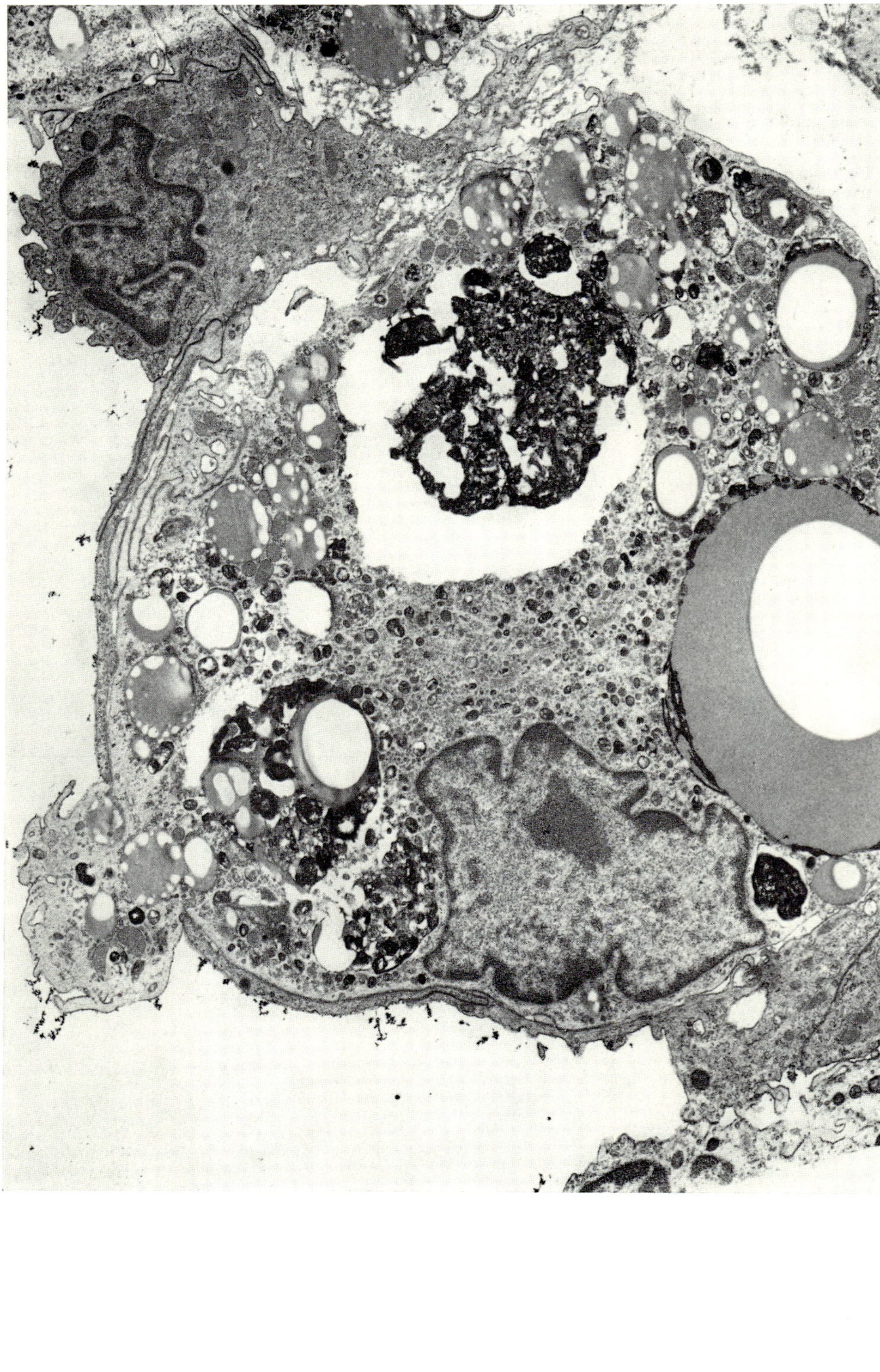

20

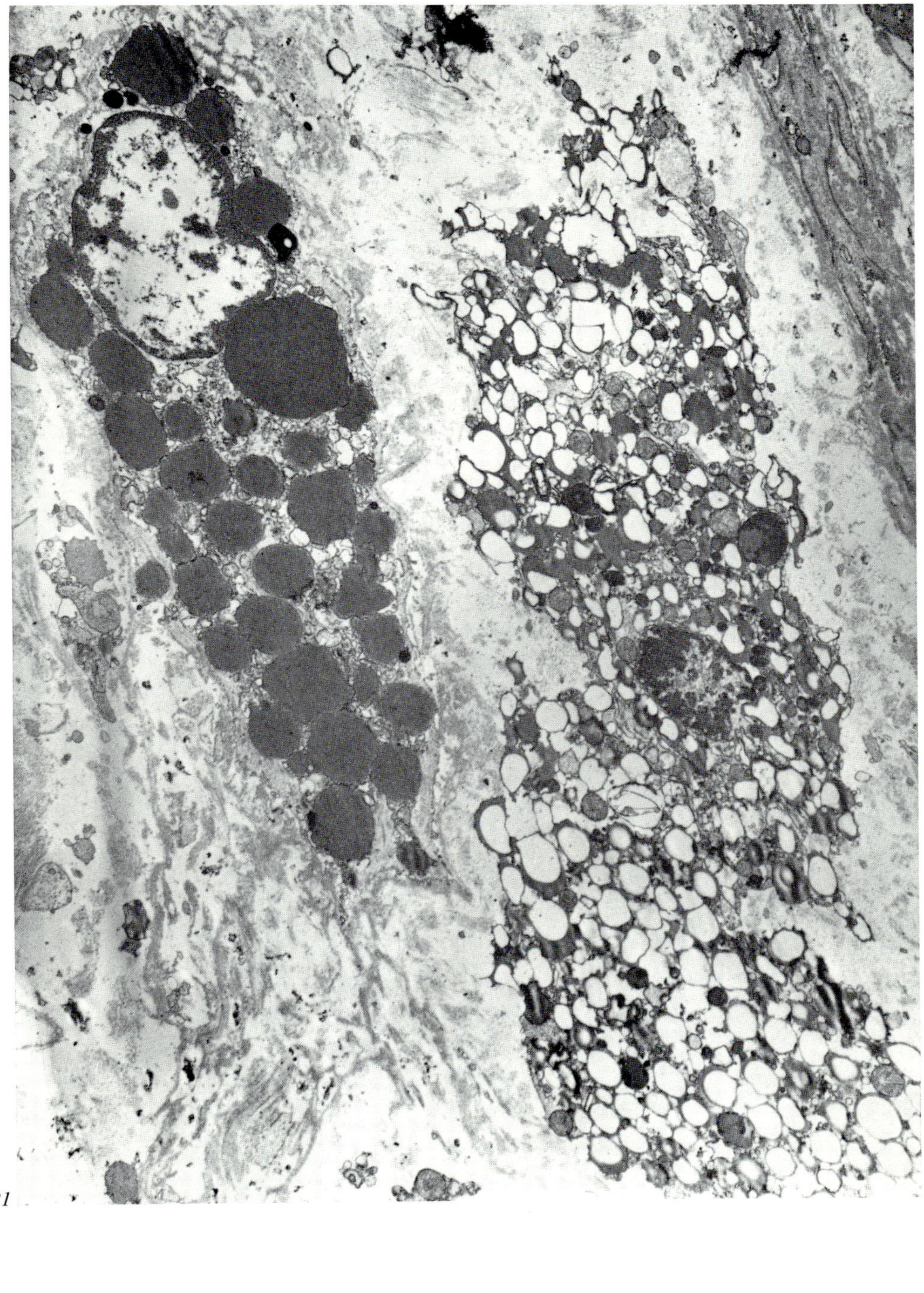

21

Page 131

Fig. 22. Aorta, descending thoracic segment, fatty streak lesion, male, age 21 years. Portion of ovoid foam cell. Note the variety of inclusions in the cytoplasm in addition to those with electron-lucid centers we identify as lipid. This cell has neither a basement membrane, micropinocytotic vesicles, nor myofilaments. Approximately $\times$ 13,500. (Reproduced with permission from GEER, J. C. and MCGILL, H. C., jr.: The evolution of the fatty streak, chapt. 2; in BREST and MOYER Atherosclerotic vascular disease. Appleton-Century-Crofts, New York 1967.)

Page 132

Fig. 23. Aorta, descending thoracic segment, fatty streak lesion, male, age 21 years. A portion of an ovoid foam cell is seen at the lower left. The cell at the upper right is a mast cell identifiable as such by the characteristic cytoplasmic inclusions. Mast cells are found in nearly all human fatty streaks in small number. Approximately $\times$ 16,000.

Page 133

Fig. 24. Aorta, descending thoracic segment, fatty streak lesion, male, age 24 years. The cells in the upper and lower portions of the micrograph are smooth muscle with lipid inclusions in the cytoplasm. The cell in the center of the micrograph cannot be identified. This cell contains numerous electron-dense granular cytoplasmic inclusions and appears to be disintegrating. The state of preservation of the cells above and below indicate that this appearance is not due to poor tissue preservation. The cell appears to be undergoing necrosis and the electron-dense granular inclusions may represent cytoplasmic degeneration. Such degeneration is one possible source of the electron-dense granular material found in the extracellular space. Approximately $\times$ 8,500.

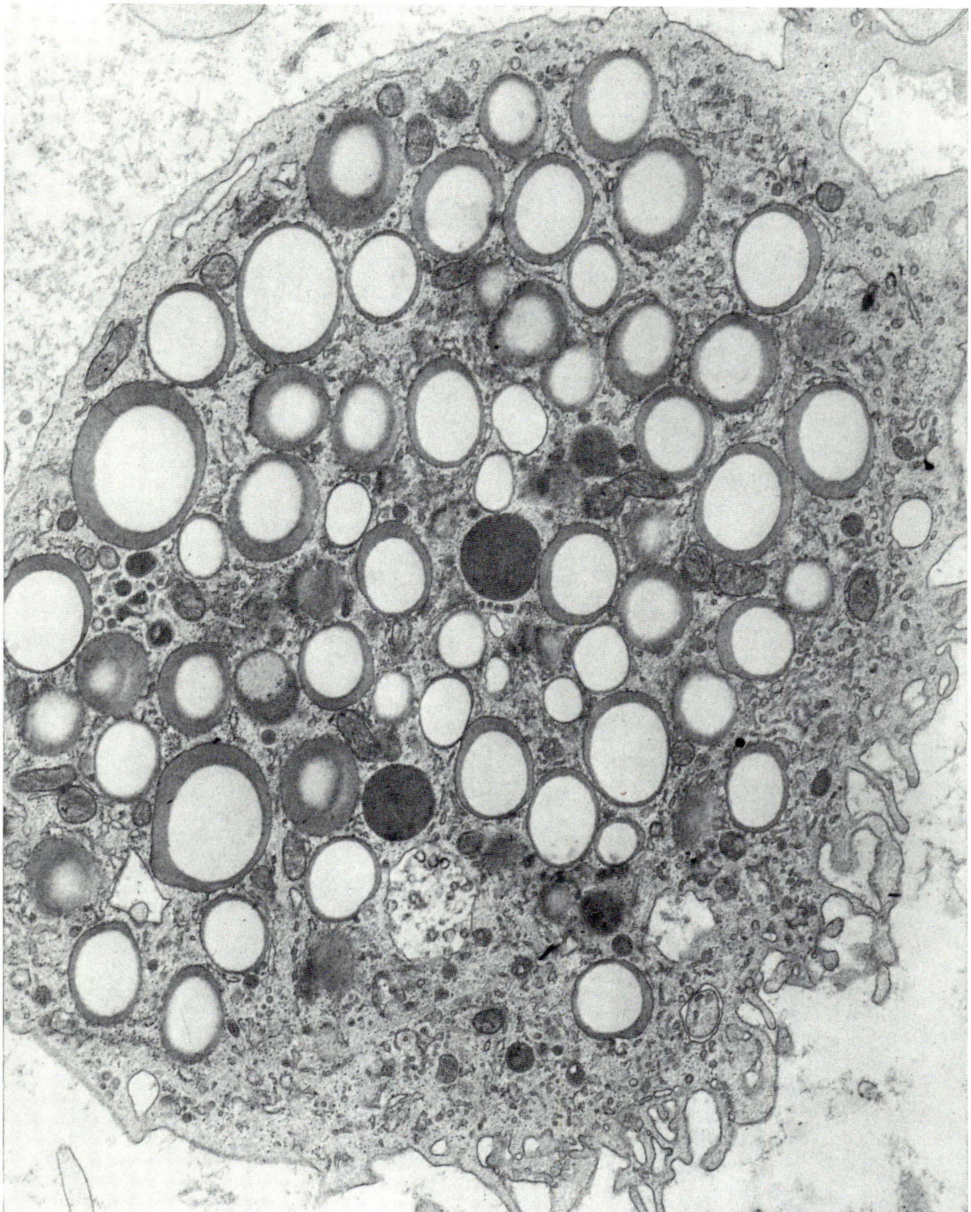

22

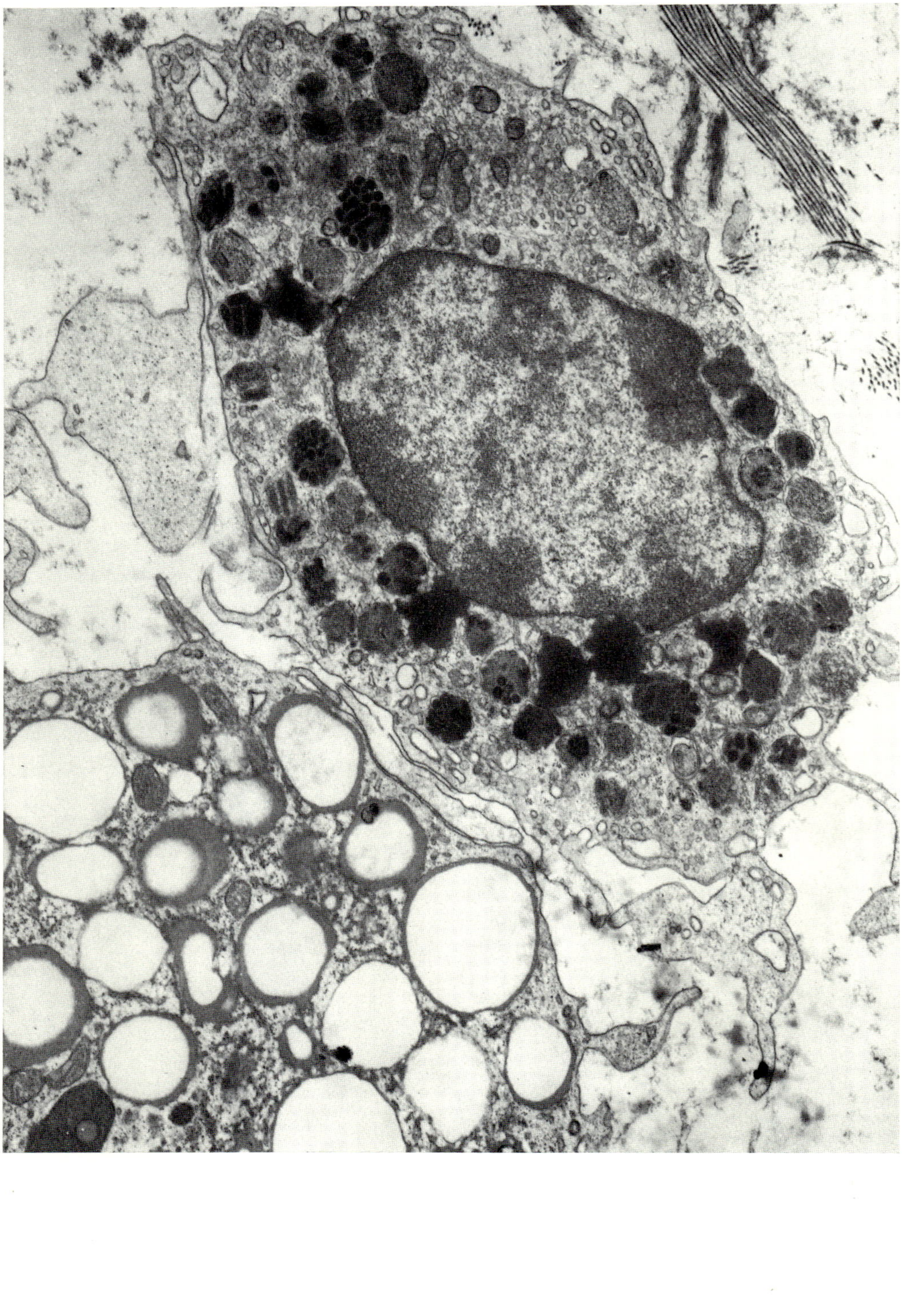

23

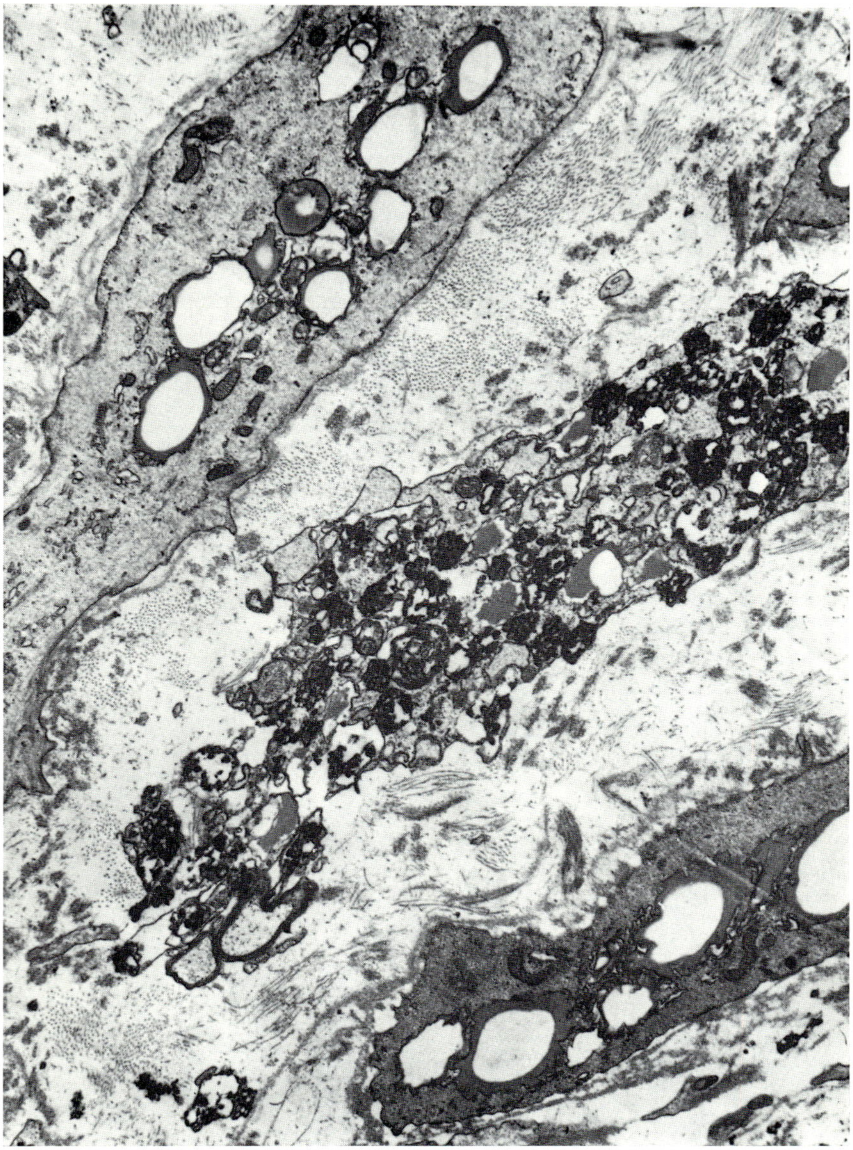

24

Page 135

Fig. 25. Coronary artery, left anterior descending branch, fibrous plaque lesion, male, age 37 years. This is a portion of a fibrous plaque lesion showing the fibrous cap on the lumen side (right), containing numerous elongated lipid-containing cells and the atheromatous core near the left margin with numerous cholesterol clefts. The junction of intima and media is just inside the left margin of the micrograph. Oil-red-O-hematoxylin stain. Approximately × 150.

Page 136

Fig. 26. Aorta, descending thoracic segment, fatty streak lesion, male, age 16 years. Though this lesion grossly appeared as a fatty streak, this cell is typical of those described in the fibrous cap of plaques and thus may be indicative of transformation of the lesion to a plaque. The cell shows numerous myofilaments among the abundant profiles of granular endoplasmic reticulum. There is abundant basement membrane material in the interstitial space with the electron-dense granular material. Approximately × 14,400.

Page 137

Fig. 27. Aorta, abdominal segment, fatty streak lesion, male, age 37 years. Among the collagen and basement membrane material in the extracellular space, there is a large amount of electron-dense granular material and an electron-lucid cleft representing a cholesterol crystal. This is the typical appearance of atheromatous debris in the core of an advanced fatty streak or a fibrous plaque. Approximately × 17,900. (Reproduced with permission from GEER, J. C.: Fine structure of human aortic intimal thickening and fatty streaks. Lab. Invest. *14:* 1764–1783, 1965.)

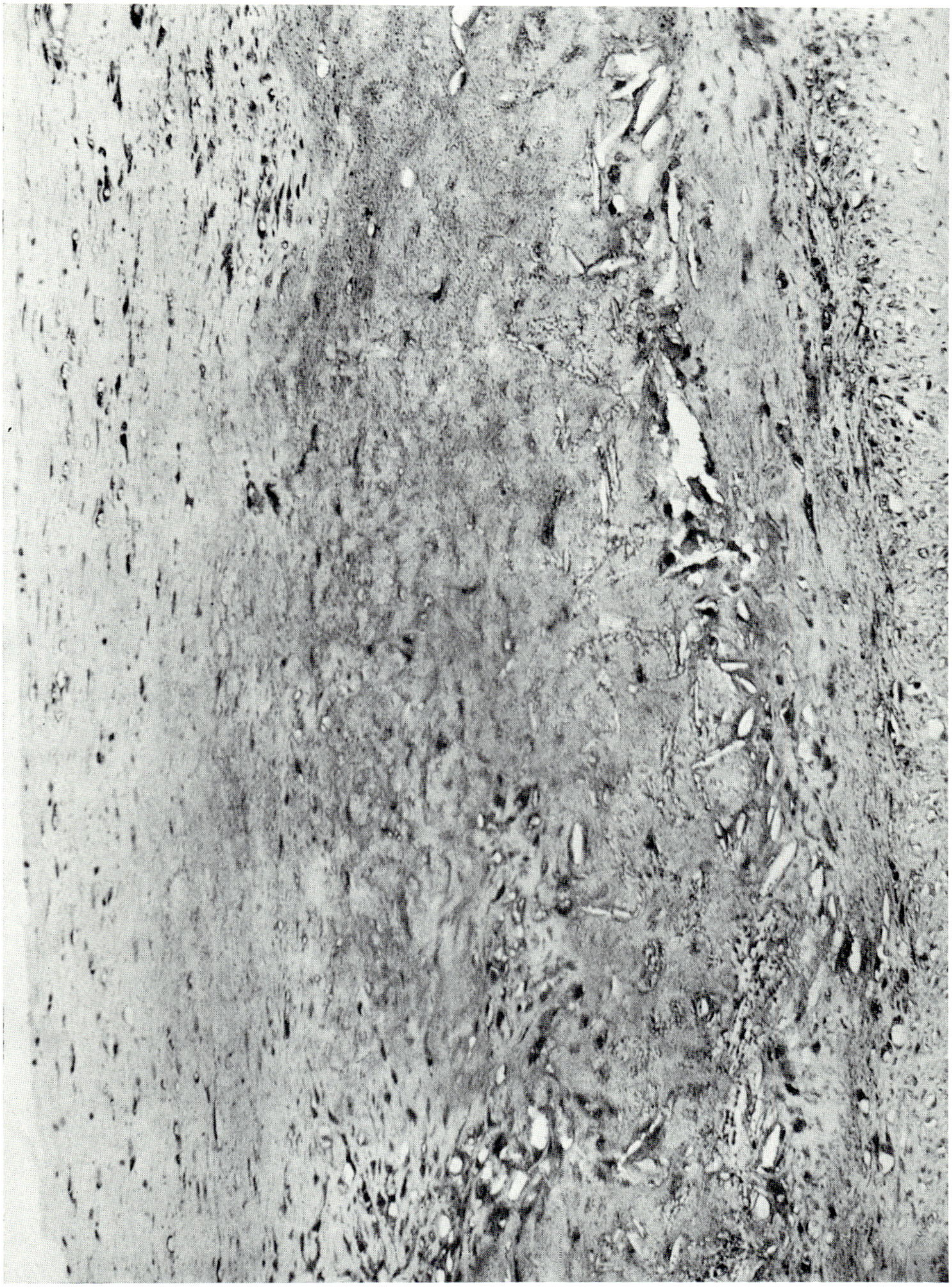

25

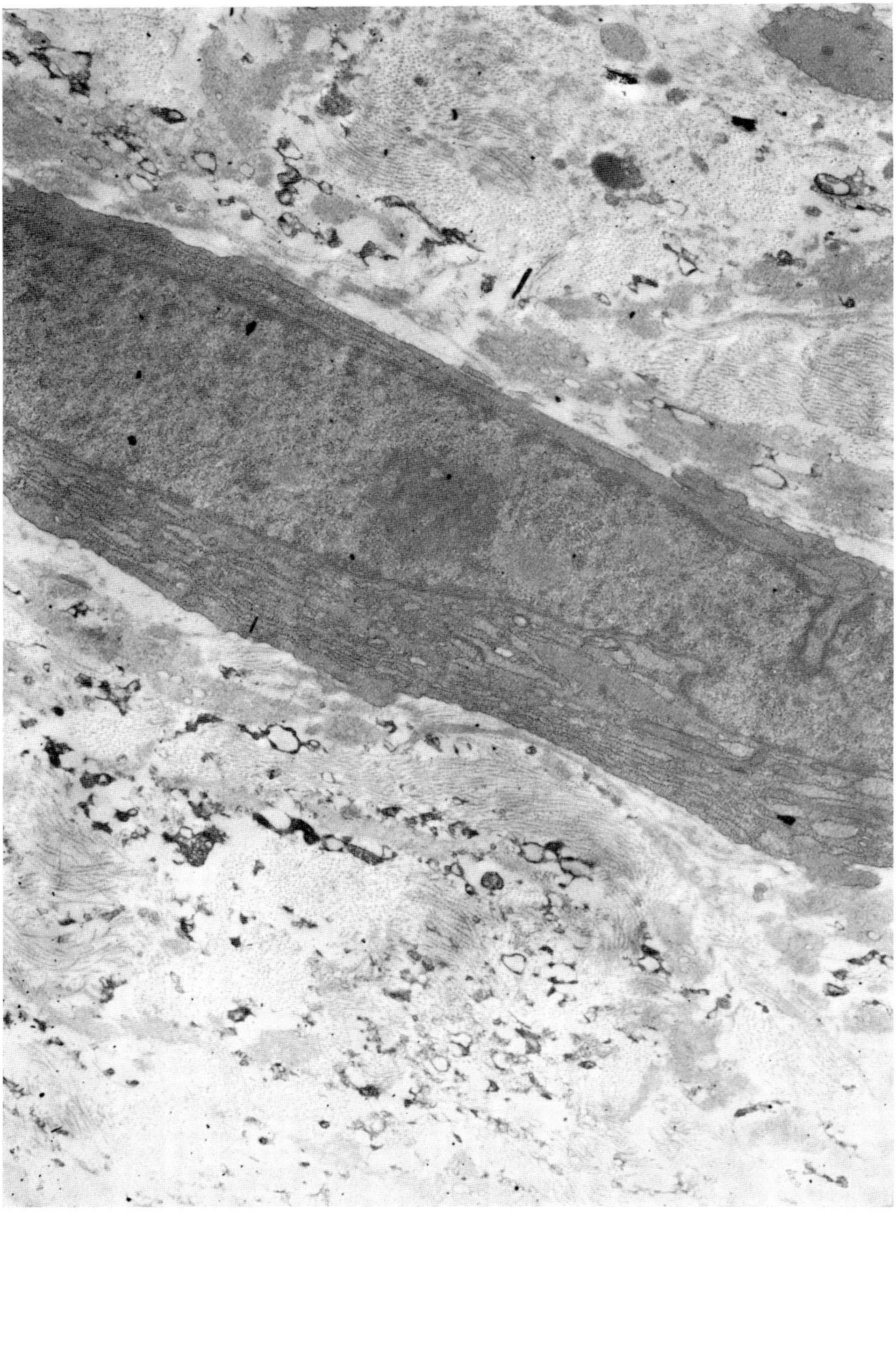

26

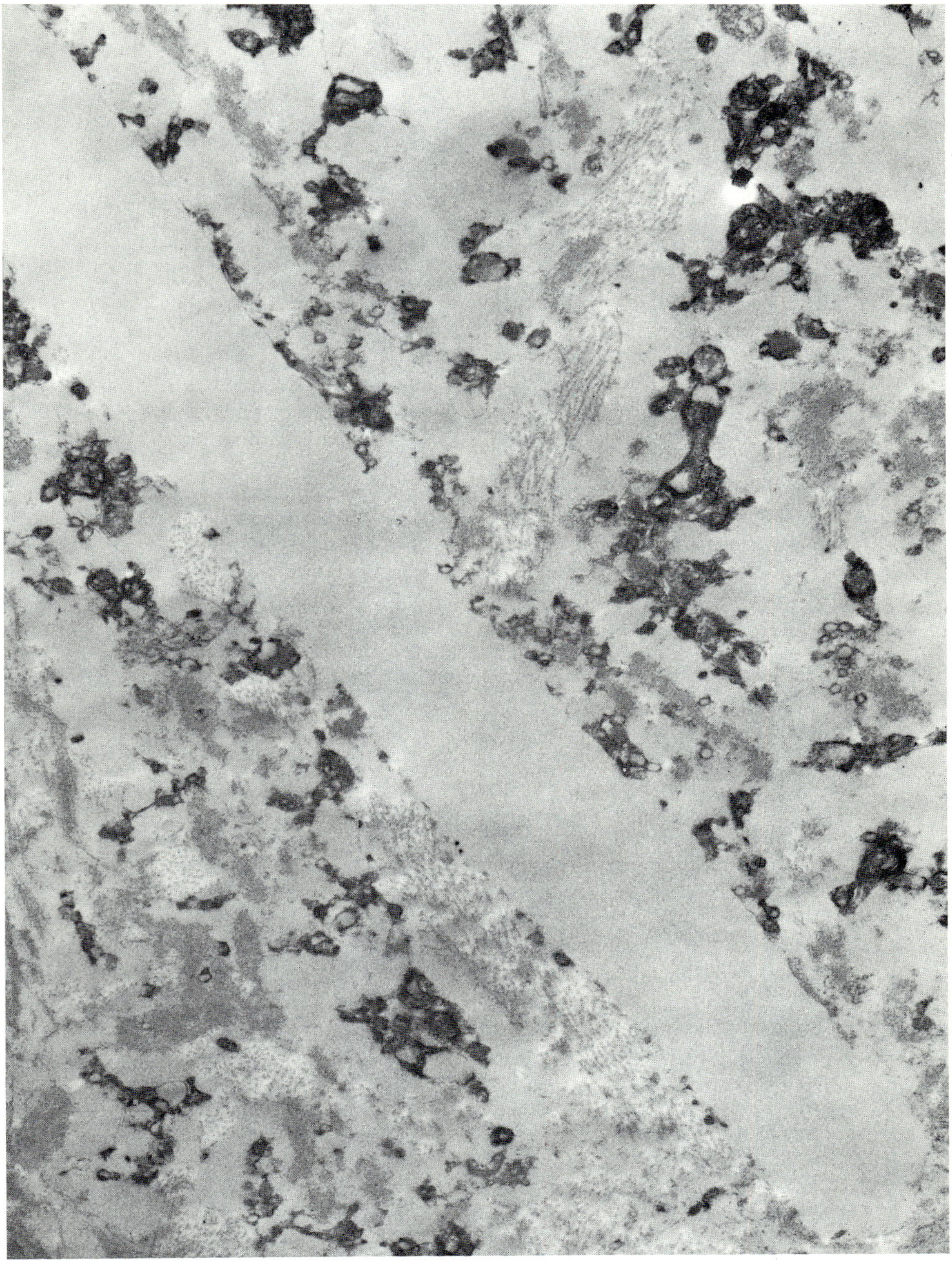

27

Subject Index